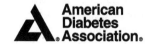

American Diabetes Association.

Practical CGM

A Guide to Improving Outcomes
through Continuous Glucose Monitoring

Gary Scheiner, MS, CDE

Director, Book Publishing, Abe Ogden; *Managing Editor,* Greg Guthrie; *Acquisitions Editor,* Victor Van Beuren; *Production Manager and Composition,* Melissa Sprott; *Copyediting,* Cenveo, Inc.; *Cover Design,* Kim Woody; *Photography,* Cameron Whitman Photography; *Printer,* United Graphics.

Printed in the United States of America

1 3 5 7 9 10 8 6 4 2

The suggestions and information contained in this publication are generally consistent with the *Standards of Medical Care in Diabetes* and other policies of the American Diabetes Association, but they do not represent the policy or position of the Association or any of its boards or committees. Reasonable steps have been taken to ensure the accuracy of the information presented. However, the American Diabetes Association cannot ensure the safety or efficacy of any product or service described in this publication. Individuals are advised to consult a physician or other appropriate health care professional before undertaking any diet or exercise program or taking any medication referred to in this publication. Professionals must use and apply their own professional judgment, experience, and training and should not rely solely on the information contained in this publication before prescribing any diet, exercise, or medication. The American Diabetes Association—its officers, directors, employees, volunteers, and members—assumes no responsibility or liability for personal or other injury, loss, or damage that may result from the suggestions or information in this publication.

Jane Chiang, MD, conducted the internal review of this book to ensure that it meets American Diabetes Association guidelines.

∞ The paper in this publication meets the requirements of the ANSI Standard Z39.48-1992 (permanence of paper).

ADA titles may be purchased for business or promotional use or for special sales. To purchase more than 50 copies of this book at a discount, or for custom editions of this book with your logo, contact the American Diabetes Association at the address below or at booksales@diabetes.org.

American Diabetes Association
1701 North Beauregard Street
Alexandria, Virginia 22311
DOI: 10.2337/9781580406031

For more information or assistance with CGM or intensive diabetes management, Gary Scheiner may be reached at (877) 735-3648 (outside North America, +1-610-642-6055) or gary@integrateddiabetes.com.

Library of Congress Cataloging-in-Publication Data

Scheiner, Gary.
  Practical continuous glucose monitoring / Gary Scheiner.
    pages cm
  Summary: "This book will help readers understand the benefits of Continuous Glucose Monitoring Systems, and how to use them properly to manage diabetes and manage it right"-- Provided by publisher.
  Includes bibliographical references and index.
  ISBN 978-1-58040-603-1 (paperback)
  1. Insulin pumps. 2. Insulin--Therapeutic use. 3. Blood sugar monitoring. I. Title.
RC661.I63S34 2015
616.4'62061--dc23
                                        2015011945

Contents

Foreword by Donna Tomky v

Foreword by Bruce Buckingham vii

Introduction. 1

1 Essentials of Continuous Glucose Monitoring 3

2 Maximizing the Benefits in Real Time 17

3 Improving Control with CGM Data Analysis 35

4 Defeating the Downsides 77

Appendix: Helpful Products for
    Sensor Site Management. 93

References 97

Index 105

Foreword

BY DONNA TOMKY

Everyone needs a practical guide to help them decipher the complex data they receive from a technological source, especially when that source is powerful continuous glucose monitoring (CGM) technology. Gary Scheiner has put together this informative and helpful guide to aid both novices and experienced practitioners in getting the best results out of CGM devices.

Practical CGM discusses who might consider using CGM devices and breaks down the particular benefits for each individual, including patients, professionals, caregivers, and significant others. Individual considerations for each device help identify which devices may be better suited for some and not for others; after all, not all devices will fit everyone perfectly! His unbiased review of the currently available CGM equipment is necessary and essential. Gary helps shed light on the performance aspects of each device and what we can expect from them. He demystifies the data that come from CGM and shows us what to do with all those numbers! Knowing what those numbers mean and how to interpret trends leads to tighter and safer glucose control. After all, isn't that what CGM is all about?

Gary is not afraid to use his own life with diabetes to illuminate the ups and downs of using a CGM device. For example, he recommends practical high-alert settings to prevent users from bolusing while insulin is on board. He appropriately calls this a "rage bolus" or an "angry bolus" when it is done in response to an apparently slow response to insulin administration. These practical and real-life examples from his life and from his practice help show that the frustration and anger many of us have experienced while using insulin are normal and understandable. What we must do is learn to work around those feelings.

CGM wearers and clinicians alike will appreciate Gary's practical guidelines for selecting useful reports and getting the best results from device software. The discussion about how to determine whether data are inaccurate or reliable is timely and important. Gary shows how statistical analysis of CGM data can guide translation of CGM data into real-life results. Through numerous examples and case studies, we see how putting information into practice can help us better interpret the complexities of CGM data. As a health-care provider, these case studies reminded me of past patients and situations that fit these patterns and made me really appreciate his brilliant insight.

Be sure to read his "Ingredients for Success," starting on page 89, which is "a series of concise best practices for CGM success." This section is a worthwhile read and perhaps should be read first to summarize how to avoid and troubleshoot problems.

Practical CGM is a practical guide for anyone using or interpreting CGM data, and I think anyone who uses CGM or helps those who use it should find this book insightful, helpful, and essential.

Donna Tomky, MSN, RN, ANP-BC, CDE, FAADE, is the 2011 Past President of the American Association of Diabetes Educators and works in the Department of Endocrinology at ABQ Health Partners in Albuquerque, NM.

Foreword

BY BRUCE BUCKINGHAM

For anyone considering using CGM—and for health-care providers who are new to or experienced with CGM use—*Practical CGM* provides a wealth of facts and tips. The principles of CGM are clearly explained and will remain valid for many years to come, even as the technology progressively improves. The current systems are explained in great detail, with many practical tips for the new or experienced user or health-care professional. This book is essential for anyone considering or currently using CGM.

One of the keys to CGM use is setting appropriate expectations. This means providing clear guidelines on how to achieve the most with a CGM and how to balance the wealth of information, which Gary appropriately calls "datus overwhelmus." Gary has done an excellent job in setting those expectations so that people using a CGM will not be overwhelmed and will be able to take full advantage of what CGM has to offer.

CGM has been available since 2000, initially for retrospective review of glucose data and then for real-time monitoring. The ability to continuously monitor glucose values was considered a game changer for diabetes management, and there were initially very high expectations about how this information would improve glycemic control and the lives of people with diabetes. These expectations are now just beginning to be realized 15 years later. The early devices were not very accurate, were bigger, and had many issues with insertion and skin reactions to adhesives. Over the last several years, there have been significant improvements in both the accuracy and the "wearability" of these devices, and they are now being integrated into consumer electronics, such as smartphones. With improved sensor accuracy, people are beginning to rely on them more and more to make diabetes-management decisions, often depending on sensor values to make insulin dose decisions "off label." *Practical CGM* acknowledges this practice and provides many helpful guidelines on how to do this safely as well as when to get an essential meter reading. Using glucose trend information in real time is critical to maximizing the benefits of a CGM. CGM users will find many examples of how to adjust their insulin boluses and manage exercise using rate-of-change information.

In the future, there will be factory-calibrated sensors that will only require the use of a meter reading when the sensor value is inconsistent with how a person is feeling. Until then, this book provides very useful guidelines for integrating meter readings with CGM devices, e.g., when to calibrate and adjust for other issues with subcutaneous sensor lag times. One of the real advantages a real-time sensor provides is the ability to generate an alarm when glucose is at a critical value or predicted to reach a critical value. This, however, is a double-edged sword since one of the major complaints with real-time sensors is the frequency of false alarms, alarm burnout, and sleep disruption for the person with diabetes and/or significant others. Gary provides helpful guidelines for getting the best results out of alarms while minimizing alarm fatigue and burnout.

Data analysis is a huge benefit for CGM users, and yet very few CGM users actually take advantage of this powerful information. I have found the information provided by CGM data analysis to be invaluable in helping people navigate the daily barriers to glycemic stability. As with daily meter glucose readings, data analysis should not be done only every three to four months at a medical appointment. This is a skill that every person with diabetes can quickly learn, and it should be practiced on a regular basis. *Practical CGM* illustrates how to use and interpret the multiple graphs and data packages provided by the CGM software. Multiple "case reports" use both the professional and personal software, and the reports cover a wide range of CGM users, including people with both type 1 and type 2 diabetes, pump and MDI (multiple daily injection) users, and people using real-time or "blinded" CGM. Even the most experienced CGM user or health-care professional can learn from these examples and begin taking full advantage of CGM data analysis.

The future vision is the integration of CGM data with insulin delivery so that the daily tasks of treatment decisions and diabetes management are reduced. Overnight glycemic control with a closed-loop system is much easier to achieve than daytime control because it does not have to deal with rapid glucose excursions due to meals and exercise. Removing the fear of prolonged nocturnal hypoglycemia and allowing a person to wake each morning with a near-normal glucose value is currently a reality that is being achieved in multiple in-home outpatient trials. Within a few years these systems may be commercially available. Hybrid closed-loop systems that rely on some user input during the day, such as meal announcement, will also be available in the next several years. These systems may give correction doses automatically based on CGM data, and the need for carbohydrate counting and diabetes "numeracy" may be removed, with only the need to announce that a meal or exercise session has been initiated. A fully closed-loop system that does not require any user input may require additional advances, such as a more rapid-acting insulin and a stable glucagon. The commercialization of these systems will be a gradually evolving process. But because these systems are *all* based on using CGM, the information Gary has provided here will continue to be useful for many years to come, even when systems that begin to "close the loop" become available.

I would recommend this book to anyone considering CGM, to experienced CGM users and to any health-care provider who is taking care of people with diabetes (whether type 1 or type 2). CGM systems are getting better and better and are becoming an integral part of managing diabetes, and *Practical CGM* offers many insights to make the best out of all that CGM offers.

Bruce Buckingham, MD, is a Professor of Pediatric Endocrinology at the Stanford School of Medicine and Stanford Children's Health.

If New Technology Falls in Our Laps, Does It Make a Sound?

It was a hot, muggy day down in southern Florida. My wife and I decided to bring the kids to visit their grandparents (aka Mom-Mom and Pop-Pop) from our home just outside of Philly. The last time we visited, we bought my parents a computer and set them up with high-speed Internet so that they could follow our blogs and video-chat with their grandkids in real time. It wasn't the best computer in the world, but it was more than good enough to surf the net and maybe even help them keep their checkbook balanced.

What we found when we arrived at their condo was not to be believed. They were using the computer, but not as we originally intended. The clock at the bottom right corner of the screen served as their bedroom clock. And they kept the screen on all the time, with a plain white background, to serve as a nightlight. Said my mom, "You think I want your father breaking a toe on his way to the bathroom in the middle of the night? The man has a prostate!"

Speaking of Mom, she also found that the edges of the display were the perfect place to leave sticky note messages for my dad. Important stuff, like "Buy eggs" and "Pick up my medication." Mom did figure out how to play solitaire on the computer, but that's the extent of their use of any actual programs. My dad found a creative use for the hardware . . . specifically, the cooling fan. They don't like running the air conditioner until the temperature reaches a thousand degrees, but that fan on the CPU, when positioned just right, could keep his legs cool while he watched TV.

I'm sharing all this unsettling information about my parents and their computer to prove a point: There is a big difference between having technology and using it to one's advantage. Continuous glucose monitoring systems (hereafter referred to as CGMs) are a perfect example. Tens of thousands of people with diabetes use CGMs, but how many are really benefiting from them? For those who are benefiting in some way, how many are taking full advantage of everything CGM has to offer? And how much are their health-care providers really able to glean from the dizzying array of data that CGMs and their accompanying software produce?

Having lived with type 1 diabetes for 30-plus years and having treated and managed clients with diabetes for more than 20 years, I've never been one to take a "woe is me" approach. We've got this disease; we'd might as well manage it right.

The purpose of this book is not to sell you on the merits of CGM. Whether you treat patients who use CGM or have diabetes (type 1 or type 2) and wear a monitor yourself, this book is all about making diabetes easier to manage. We're past the point of being in awe of CGM's cool-looking graphics. It's time to start reaping the benefits of this innovative technology. Technology to benefit us all.

To communicate effectively with CGM users and clinicians worldwide, glucose data throughout this book will be expressed in both mg/dL and mmol/L. The mmol/L values will be placed in square brackets. For example, 180 [10] means 180 mg/dL or 10 mmol/L.

CHAPTER 1

Essentials of Continuous Glucose Monitoring

There's a reason so many major companies have invested heavily in fingerstick glucose monitoring. Point-in-time glucose readings are valuable, and not just for those who are pricking their fingers. They rake in *billions* for medical device manufacturers because they allow us to titrate (fine-tune) insulin and medication doses, see cause-and-effect relationships within our daily lives, conduct cutting-edge research on new treatments, and fix elements of diabetes management programs that just aren't working. Like a photograph or a painting, fingerstick blood glucose (BG) readings depict what is happening at a particular moment in time, but they also leave a lot to the imagination. Take any 10 people and show them a portrait of da Vinci's *Mona Lisa*, and you'll hear 10 different interpretations about who she was, what she was like, and what she was thinking about.

As we will discuss in Chapter 2, adding a continuous glucose monitor (CGM) to one's diabetes management is like taking all those images and turning them into a movie, complete with "story notes." CGM lets us see and understand the full picture—where we came from, where we are, and to an extent, where we're headed. CGM's alert features provide the user with an early warning system to guard against severe hypoglycemia and prolonged hyperglycemia. And the ability to analyze CGM data retrospectively gives health-care providers and their patients an opportunity to make decisions based on facts rather than assumptions.

These are among the reasons that CGM is growing in popularity. There is no question that the technology still has considerable room for improvement, and our ability to interpret CGM data is still evolving. Nevertheless, CGM has already been shown to be an effective tool for improving glucose control and quality of life for users.[1-5]

GET TO KNOW THE EQUIPMENT

Currently, Dexcom and Medtronic offer CGM systems in the United States. Although systems by other manufacturers are available in other countries, our discussions will focus on devices that are approved by the U.S. Food and Drug Administration (FDA) and available for sale in the U.S. In addition to *real-time* systems that allow the user to see, learn from, and react to their own data, both Medtronic and Dexcom offer *professional use* systems. Professional systems are borrowed for a fixed period of time (typically 6–7 days). The only significant difference between systems is whether the user is able to see their data while they wear the sensor. The Dexcom G4 Professional system has an option that allows the user to see their data in real time or to blind it (not showing it on the display) until the receiver is downloaded. The Medtronic Professional system, called iPro, is always blinded to the user. Health-care providers download the professional system after removing the sensor from the patient and analyze the information to make therapy adjustments.

Regardless of the manufacturer and whether the device is for real-time or professional use, three components are common to all CGM systems: a sensor, a transmitter, and a receiver or display.

Sensors

The *sensor* is a thin, flexible, metallic filament that is about a finger-width long (Fig. 1.1). It is placed in the layer of fat below the skin using a push-button *insertion device* (Fig. 1.2). The insertion device pops a small needle (with the sensor attached) into the skin and then retracts the needle, leaving only the sensor below the skin. The insertion process is virtually painless when done properly; training by a device manufacturer representative is highly recommended. Sensors are indicated for ~1 week of use (6 days for the Medtronic Enlite; 7 days for the Dexcom G4). Anecdotally, users have reported the ability to use sensors for longer than their FDA-approved indication, but at present no controlled studies have evaluated the safety and efficacy of prolonged sensor use.

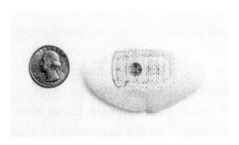

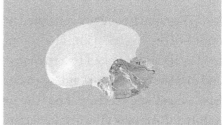

Figure 1.1—Sensors.

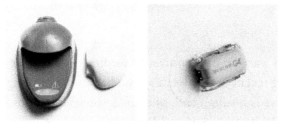

Figure 1.2—Insertion devices.

TRANSMITTERS

Once below the skin, the sensor reacts with glucose molecules by generating a miniscule electric current. This current travels up to the base of the sensor on the skin surface where it connects to a *transmitter* (Fig. 1.3). The transmitter is about the size of a thumbnail. It contains its own power source and a radio transmitter. Transmitters require periodic charging or replacement to keep the power fresh.

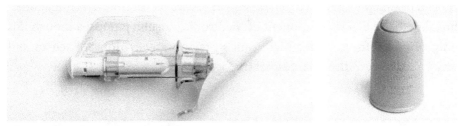

Figure 1.3—Transmitters. The image on the left also shows the transmitter charger.

Receivers and Displays

The radio frequency generated by the transmitter varies based on the magnitude of the electrical impulse coming from the sensor. Each transmitter has a unique ID and is linked to a *receiver*—a device that interprets the radio signals and displays the corresponding glucose data (Fig. 1.4). The Dexcom CGM utilizes a handheld receiver about the size of a small cellular phone. It also transmits to the Animas Vibe insulin pump and soon will be able to transmit to other insulin pumps. The Medtronic CGM display is integrated into Medtronic insulin pumps (model x22 and higher). Medtronic also offers a stand-alone receiver (not an insulin pump) called Guardian. The Guardian receiver has similar functionality to the CGM component of Medtronic's insulin pumps, although it is only approved for use with Medtronic's previous-generation Sof-sensor and uses an older algorithm to interpret the signals.

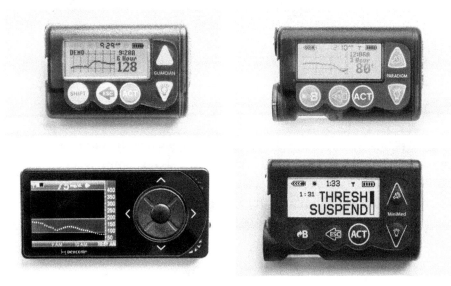

Figure 1.4—Receivers and displays.

CGM receivers display a variety of important *real-time information*, including trend graphs covering recent time intervals; trend arrows indicating the current direction the glucose is headed; and, of course, the latest glucose value generated by the sensor. Both Medtronic and Dexcom receivers provide updated information every 5 min. The receivers also emit audible and vibratory *alerts.* Users and their clinicians can customize the alert settings to suit individual preferences and achieve specific goals. Alert options include the following:

◆ Basic high and low alerts—as soon as the sensor detects a glucose concentration that has crossed a user-set threshold, an alert is triggered

◆ Rate-of-change alerts—any time the glucose concentration is rising or falling faster than a user-set rate, an alert is triggered

◆ Predictive alerts—these alerts incorporate aspects of both the high/low and rate-of-change alerts. If the glucose concentration is *expected* to cross a user-set high/low threshold in a relatively short period of time based on the current glucose and rate of change, an alert is triggered. This feature is only available on Medtronic systems.

A Medtronic 530G insulin pump can temporarily suspend basal insulin delivery when a low threshold is crossed. The next-generation pump-sensor combination will have the ability to reduce or suspend basal delivery to *prevent* hypoglycemia. And plans are already underway for more automated modes of glucose regulation, including the prevention of both high and low glucose levels based on sensor glucose (SG) values and trends.

Receivers are utilized for another vital role: calibration. The timely entry of accurate fingerstick BG values is necessary to keep the sensor working properly and to maximize its accuracy. More details regarding optimal calibration will be presented in Chapter 4.

Medtronic and Dexcom offer *software* for downloading and displaying data from CGM receivers. Medtronic's CareLink software allows CGM users and their health-care providers to download and access CGM (and corresponding pump) data on a web-based platform. CareLink Pro is an office-based software housed on individual computers. It provides more detailed reports than Care-Link, along with some pattern analysis.

Dexcom's Studio software is a PC-based program that generates a variety of reports specific to the CGM and any events entered by the user. Data files and individual reports can be shared between patients and clinicians via e-mail. A limited number of open-platform web-based programs, such as Diasend, allow Dexcom users to integrate their CGM data with certain insulin pumps and BG meters.

We'll discuss much more about the components and features of the various CGM software programs when we explore data reports in Chapter 3.

Both Medtronic and Dexcom also offer *ancillary transmission equipment* for sending CGM data over a distance to caregivers and loved ones. Medtronic's mySentry (Fig. 1.5) is an alarm clock of sorts that parents and caregivers can use to track a loved one's CGM data from another room. mySentry includes a signal amplifier that sits near the person who is wearing the CGM, and a table-top display that sits in another room. The remote display provides the same information as the usual CGM display, and can be set to emit a powerful alarm in the event of a glucose control or sensor performance issue.

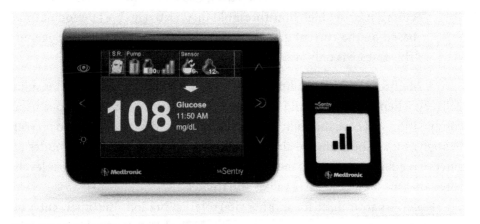

Figure 1.5—Medtronic mySentry receiver, display, and signal transmitter.

Dexcom recently introduced the SHARE device and G4 SHARE receiver. The SHARE device is essentially a cradle that takes data from the Dexcom receiver and transmits it via Bluetooth to a mobile device (iPhone, iPod Touch) so that the data can be transmitted to Dexcom's cloud-based server (Fig. 1.6). This data, in turn, can be displayed on the iPhone or iPod Touch of a person who has been invited to "follow" the Dexcom user. The person following the data can also receive alerts on their mobile device when glucose alerts are taking place. Free apps must be installed on the transmitting and receiving devices for the system to work, but it allows the tracking of a loved one's sensor data from virtually anywhere in the world. The G4 SHARE receiver eliminates the need for the cradle. Its built-in Bluetooth device transmits data directly to an iPhone or iPod Touch (Fig. 1.7).

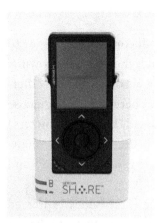

Figure 1.6—Dexcom SHARE transmission cradle.

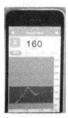

Figure 1.7—Dexcom SHARE follower app.

Because Dexcom's SHARE system requires two smart devices and is not readily portable if the cradle is used (it is tethered to a power outlet), many Dexcom users—particularly parents of children with type 1 diabetes—use a program called NightScout—sometimes referred to as "CGM in the Cloud." With this program, the Dexcom receiver is connected directly to a portable Android phone that transmits data to a cloud-based server. Individuals with the proper link may access the data on their mobile device. Note that NightScout was designed and is made available by tech-savvy parents of children with diabetes. It is not FDA approved and is not supported by Dexcom (full details and instructions can be found at www.nightscout.info).

PERFORMANCE

CGM systems are far from ideal. Their accuracy is still considered inferior to fingerstick testing (using up-to-date meters), although the gap is narrowing. In most circles, CGM accuracy is measured by mean absolute relative difference percentage (MARD%), or the average discrepancy between CGM glucose values and simultaneous capillary BG values (taken with fingerstick meters) or venous serum glucose (via laboratory equipment, better known as a Yellow Springs Instrument [YSI]). Fingerstick meter values are generally within 5 and 10% of YSI, whereas CGM is generally within 10 and 20%.

To understand MARD%, consider this example (first values expressed in mg/dL; values in square brackets expressed in mmol/L). We first take the difference between the value obtained on a meter or CGM and the lab value taken at the same time, and then we divide this difference by the lab value to determine the *percent* difference between the obtained value and the lab value. This is the percent the obtained value was "off by." We then average these "off by" values to obtain our MARD% (see example in Table 1.1).

Table 1.1—Example: Calculating Average Percent Difference

Meter (or CGM) value (mg/dL [mmol/L])	Simultaneous lab glucose value (mg/dL [mmol/L])	Absolute difference (mg/dL [mmol/L])	Percent difference (absolute difference ÷ lab value) (%)
158 [8.78]	177 [9.83]	19 [1.05]	11
73 [4.06]	62 [3.44]	11 [0.62]	18
244 [13.56]	222 [12.33]	22 [1.23]	10
185 [10.28]	170 [9.44]	15 [0.84]	9
99 [5.50]	113 [6.28]	14 [0.78]	12
Average percent difference (MARD%):			12

MARD%, mean absolute relative difference percentage.

Some CGM systems produce better accuracy than others, and each company's next-generation system leaves previous versions in the dust (see Table 1.2).

Table 1.2—Comparison of Medtronic Enlite versus Dexcom GM Systems

System	MARD% (vs. meter capillary glucose)	MARD% (vs. laboratory— Yellow Springs Instrument or HemoCue)	User guide specifications (vs. YSI)
Medtronic (Enlite)	19.9% [6]	18% [10]	14.0% [12,*]
	16.7% [7]	16.6% [6]	16.7% [13,#]
	18.9% [8]	17.9% [11]	
	17.8% [9]	17.5% [7]	
		16.4% [8]	
		17.8% [9]	
Dexcom (G4)	12.2% [6]	13.6% [6]	13.3% [15,#]
	10.9% [13]	10.8% [11]	11.3% [14,‡]
	13.9% [9]	13.9% [9]	
		9.0% [14,‡]	

*Calibration performed three to four times daily; #calibration performed twice daily; ‡using algorithm introduced November 2014.

Sources: Adapted from Kropff et al.[6]; Freckmann et al.[7]; Luijf et al.[8]; Matuleviciene et al.[9]; Calhoun et al.[10]; Damiano et al.[11]; Medtronic[12]; Pleus et al.[13]; Bailey et al.[14]; Dexcom.[15]

LAG TIME AND INACCURACY

There is a catch, however. Whereas fingerstick (capillary) glucose readings are current—they represent the glucose concentration at that exact moment—CGM data has some lag time. It's like watching a breaking news report about an event that took place 10 min ago. Useful to know, but it's not quite like being there when it happened.

There are two reasons for the lag. First, CGM sensors are not measuring BG directly. They are measuring the glucose concentration in the fluid surrounding fat cells below the skin, and it takes some time for glucose to diffuse (travel) from the blood into those tissues. When the BG concentration is rising, it may take a few minutes for the extra glucose to show up in the fat layer. And when it is falling, it will take several minutes for the reduction to take place in the fat layer.

A second reason for the delayed measurement is the way CGMs process data. They receive continuous radio signals from the transmitter that is connected to the sensor, yet most CGMs provide updated numeric values and trend graph reports every 5 min. They take the data received over the 5-min period, lop off potentially erroneous values, and average the rest. So new values displayed on the receiver are an average of 2.5 min old. This information remains on screen for another 5 min until another update appears, so the data being displayed is anywhere from 2.5 to 7.5 min old.

Lag time, which has been estimated to range from ~6 to 12 min,[16-18] has important implications. When BG levels are rising, the CGM is likely to display values that are *lower* than the actual BG. And when it is falling, the CGM is likely to display values that are *higher* than the actual BG. Knowing this allows for more appropriate interpretation of CGM data, better calibration technique, and setting of appropriate expectations on the part of both the user and clinician (Fig. 1.8).

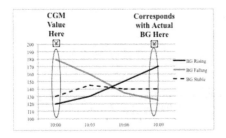

| | Corresponds with | | | |
CGM value at	fingerstick value at	If BG is rising	If BG is falling	If BG is stable
10:10 a.m.	9:58–10:04 a.m.	CGM is probably lower than the fingerstick	CGM is probably higher than the fingerstick	CGM and fingerstick should be similar

Figure 1.8—Example lag time.

A significant part of CGM's inaccuracy can be traced to lag time and the fact that the sensors are not measuring BG directly. Other factors contributing to inaccuracy include improper sensor insertion, skin irritation (sometimes caused by sensor movement or trauma to the site), and suboptimal calibration practices.

All CGM systems require calibration by way of fingerstick glucose entries. Calibrations typically are required two or three times daily. Untimely calibration entries, use of an unreliable meter, or improper BG-monitoring technique on the part of the user will affect sensor accuracy and performance. When sensor accuracy is poor, high and low alerts may be triggered inappropriately (false positives), or alerts may not be triggered at times when they should be (false negatives). When calibration values deviate significantly from sensor values on a repeated basis, the CGM system will sometimes generate alarms or terminate the sensor session completely. We will discuss techniques for improving sensor accuracy in Chapter 4.

Despite these issues, sensor accuracy has improved considerably over the past several years. MARD, system complexity, and the incidence of errors have been greatly reduced. Those who tried and abandoned a previous-generation CGM because of performance issues should be encouraged to try the latest systems.

MAINTENANCE

Another aspect of CGM use involves routine maintenance. The sensors are the main disposable item in the system. Each manufacturer's sensors have an approved duration of usage. The receiver will alert the user when it is time to change the sensor. This may occur earlier than expected if the sensor is not performing properly.

Keeping sensors in place and stable requires adequate adhesion. Although adhesive aids on the skin surface are discouraged because of their potential to interact with the sensor's delicate chemistry, over-bandages and under-bandages are widely used. In our experience, the use of extra adhesive products has little to no detrimental effect on sensor performance.

In terms of electrical power, transmitters and receivers require routine maintenance. Medtronic CGM systems require AAA battery changes in the receiver (insulin pump or Guardian) every 2–3 weeks, and the MiniLink and iPro transmitters must be charged after every 6 days of use. The device that charges the MiniLink transmitter also uses a disposable AAA battery that requires periodic replacement. The MiniLink and iPro transmitters may be recharged many times but will not last forever; they typically require replacement on at least an annual basis.

Dexcom's receiver requires recharging every 5–7 days via plug-in to a wall outlet, computer, or car's AC port. The Dexcom transmitter never requires charging, but usually needs to be replaced 9–12 months after removal from its original packaging.

WHO IS IT GOOD FOR?

In the chapters that follow, we will take a close look at the value to be derived from CGM usage. We'll also present proven strategies for overcoming system shortcomings and explore experience-based techniques for optimizing the benefit from CGM systems. Given that a cost-to-benefit ratio is involved in using CGM and that health-care resources are limited, it is worth taking a look at who are the most appropriate candidates for CGM.

Upon its inception more than a decade ago, CGM was viewed as an elite item only to be used in exceptional cases. Today, with considerable improvements in usability and performance as well as expanded private insurance coverage, CGM can play a role in improving the care and management of a significant portion of the diabetes population. Health professional organizations[19–22] recommend CGM usage for adults and children who use insulin, particularly those who—

> Given the multitude of ways in which CGM can be utilized, it may be more practical to screen those who are *not* appropriate candidates rather than searching for those who are.

- ◆ Check their BG regularly and are committed to intensive diabetes management
- ◆ Have hypoglycemia unawareness or frequent hypoglycemia[1]
- ◆ Experience considerable variability in BG levels
- ◆ Require an HbA_{1c} reduction without increased hypoglycemia[1]
- ◆ Are planning or entering a change in therapy, such as initiating multiple-daily-injection or insulin-pump therapy[2]
- ◆ Participate in sports or athletics
- ◆ Engage in a high-risk professions and need to ensure avoidance of hypoglycemia

Although not formally tested or FDA approved for use during pregnancy, CGM use has been associated with improved glycemic control, lower birth weight, and reduced risk of macrosomia.[3] In light of rapidly changing insulin requirements, the need to maintain very tight glucose control (particularly during postprandial phases), and the risk of severe hypoglycemia, we have found that CGM can serve as a valuable management tool throughout pregnancy.

In addition, CGM can be helpful for those who do not use insulin.[4,5] Potential applications include the following:

♦ Titrating medication doses
♦ Intensifying medical therapy
♦ Uncovering behaviors that may be influencing glycemic control positively or negatively
♦ Teaching cause-and-effect relationships between lifestyle choices and glycemic control

CHAPTER 2

Maximizing the Benefits in Real Time

N ow let's turn our attention to what we all came for: *What the heck can we get out of these devices?* This section explores the benefits a user can experience from using CGM data in real time.

REAL TIME, REAL BENEFITS

Like my kids (or The Tops or Calling Birds), really good things come in fours. And there are four distinct benefits to be derived from CGM in real time:

◆ Use of the numbers
◆ Trending information
◆ High/low alerts
◆ Pump integration

Benefit 1. Use of the Numbers

First, consider the glucose values themselves. Medtronic and Dexcom CGM systems display an updated glucose value every 5 min. The values are based on averaged data collected over the previous 5-min time period, with potentially erroneous values deleted.

Remember, these aren't exactly *BG* concentrations. They are interstitial-fluid-between-the-fat-cells glucose concentrations. Although these values correlate closely with BG, there are some differences, most notably lag time as discussed in Chapter 1. As such, most regulatory bodies (including the FDA) have not approved CGM as a replacement for fingerstick glucose measurements.

Is it really so bad that the SG values differ from the meter-derived BG values? Remember, in keeping with current International Organization for Standardization standards, most modern BG meters vary from laboratory values by 5–10%, and older meters vary by 10–20%. The fact is, when functioning properly, CGMs are not far off from meters when it comes to accuracy.

Despite product label warnings to the contrary, users of CGM systems often use the displayed glucose values for decision-making purposes *without* confirmatory fingersticks. Although not an approved or recommended practice, there are some potential advantages to doing this. For those who historically perform fewer than the number of daily fingersticks recommended by their health-care providers, CGM provides *some* basis for decision making when it comes to food, exercise, and insulin or other medication doses. For those who are used to checking their BG more than four times per day, use of CGM may help to cut down on the cost, inconvenience, discomfort, and waste associated with excessive fingerstick procedures.

From a health care provider standpoint, it is important to recognize and accept that CGM users engage in this practice (just like underage people sometimes consume alcohol) and guide patients appropriately. We never *recommend* using SG values for calculating insulin doses, but if a CGM user chooses to do so, it is best that they do so as responsibly as possible. The trustworthiness of the SG must be considered. Specifically, the following conditions should be met before using SG values to make critical decisions:

1. The user has experience using CGM. For most people, it takes three or four sensor lifecycles before the nuances of the system are well understood. In other words, don't trust the data if you are a CGM newbie.
2. The sensor has been generating data for at least 12–24 h. During the first 12–24 h of use, SG tends to be considerably less accurate than it will become later on. It takes a few calibrations and formation of a stable wound at the sensor site for the system to home in and become reliable.

3. The last couple of calibration (fingerstick) values have matched the sensor values reasonably well, with <15% discrepancies. Say what you will about the accuracy of BG versus SG. If the SG is way off from the meter, I'd go with the meter values.

4. The current glucose is not rising or falling rapidly. This is a lag-time issue. When rising, SG tends to be lower than BG, and when falling, SG tends to be higher. There's simply too much chance of applying a grossly inaccurate value when the glucose is in a state of flux. As a general rule, if there are up (↑,↗) or down (↓,↘) arrows on the display, best to take a fingerstick reading to obtain a more current glucose value.

5. You are not recovering from hypoglycemia. To see whether your glucose level has returned to a safe range after treating a low, only use fingerstick values. Lag time, combined with the fact that blood flow to the skin surface (and the layer of fat below the skin surface) is often blunted in a state of hypoglycemia, produces artificially low SG values for up to 30–60 min. Trusting the CGM under these conditions may lead to overtreatment of the low and subsequent high glucose levels.

6. Interfering substances (such as acetaminophen, with the Dexcom system) have not been utilized for a reasonable period of time.

Benefit 2. Applying The Trend

Next, let's take a look at the trending information. *Trending* refers to whether the SG is stable, rising, or falling. There are two ways to identify trends: on-screen direction arrows and trend graphs.

The images in Fig. 2.1 were taken from a couple of old-school CGM systems, but the point still applies to the latest devices on the market.

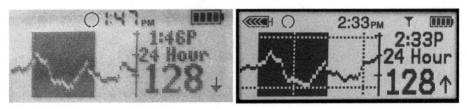

Fig. 2.1*A*   Fig. 2.1*B*

Figure 2.1—Two CGM displays: same number; different directions.

Both Fig. 2.1*A* and Fig. 2.1*B* show identical SG values, 128 mg/dL [7.1 mmol/L]. The difference is the direction the glucose is headed. In the trend graph in Fig. 2.1*A*, the glucose is falling; in Fig. 2.1*B*, it is rising.

Each system attaches its own definitions to the trend arrows associated with a recent change in glucose values (Table 2.1).

Table 2.1—Trend Arrows

	Medtronic	Dexcom
	In the past 20 min:	In the past 15 min:
→	n/a	SG changing <1 mg/dL/min [0.06 mmol/L]
↗	n/a	SG rising 1–2 mg/dL/min [0.06–0.11 mmol/L]
↑	SG rising 1–2 mg/dL/min [0.06–0.11 mmol/L]	SG rising 2–3 mg/dL/min [0.11–0.17 mmol/L]
↑↑	SG rising >2 mg/dL/min [0.11 mmol/L]	SG rising >3 mg/dL/min [0.17 mmol/L]
↘	n/a	SG falling 1–2 mg/dL/min [0.06–0.11 mmol/L]
↓	SG falling 1–2 mg/dL/min [0.06–0.11 mmol/L]	SG falling 2–3 mg/dL/min [0.11–0.17 mmol/L]
↓↓	SG falling >2 mg/dL/min [0.11 mmol/L]	SG rising >3 mg/dL/min [0.17 mmol/L]

n/a, not applicable; SG, sensor glucose.

Decision Making

Why is it important to know what direction the glucose is going? Simply put, it helps users to make smarter decisions. Knowing the direction (and not just the current value) allows users to predict, with reasonable accuracy, where their glucose level will be for the next 30–60 min.

When would this be important? How about before exercise? A quick glance at the CGM receiver can let a user know the best course of action for optimizing glucose control during the activity. Consider this example: Jenny receives basal insulin from her insulin pump. She is getting ready for her 5 P.M. aerobics class and normally takes a small snack (10–15 g carb) before the workout to prevent hypoglycemia if her BG is near normal. A quick look at her CGM, however, lets her know the direction her glucose level is headed and gives her a better idea of what she needs to do (Table 2.2).

Table 2.2—Jenny's CGM

Pre-exercise BG	Usual course of action	Sensor direction	Optimal course of action
125 mg/dL [6.9 mmol/L]	Take 10–15 g carb before exercise	➜ (stable)	Take 10–15 g carb before exercise
125 mg/dL [6.9 mmol/L]	Take 10–15 g carb before exercise	↘, ↓ (falling modestly)	Take 20–30 g carb before exercise
125 mg/dL [6.9 mmol/L]	Take 10–15 g carb before exercise	↓↓ (falling rapidly)	Take 30–40 g carb; wait 15 min and recheck BG before exercising
125 mg/dL [6.9 mmol/L]	Take 10–15 g carb before exercise	↗, ↑ (rising modestly)	Okay to exercise; no snack necessary
125 mg/dL [6.9 mmol/L]	Take 10–15 g carb before exercise	↑↑ (rising rapidly)	Okay to exercise; check BG in 15–20 min; administer insulin bolus if markedly elevated

Similarly, knowing the direction SG is headed can prove valuable when preparing for these situations:

- Taking a quiz, test, or examination
- Driving an automobile
- Using industrial equipment
- Going to sleep
- Undergoing a medical procedure
- Delivering a performance or presentation
- Heading into important meetings
- Engaging in sexual activity

In many situations, a normal SG that is dropping signals the need for extra carbohydrates, whereas a normal glucose that is rising might require extra insulin or physical activity to keep the glucose within a normal range. A follow-up glucose check in the next 30–60 min also would be in order for a timely update.

Hypoglycemia Treatment

Knowing the direction the glucose is headed (and rate of change) can aid in proper treatment of hypoglycemia. Simply put, there are garden-variety lows—episodes that can be treated in a standard manner—and there are hell-bent lows that require extra-aggressive treatment. We have found it helpful to look at the shape and direction of the trend graph when deciding on the best way to handle a low (Table 2.3).

Table 2.3—Trend Patterns and Adjustments

Current trend graph pattern	Adjustment to hypoglycemia treatment
Dropping only slightly	Treat with usual amount of carbohydrate
Falling in a steady manner	Add 25% to the usual treatment amount
Accelerating downward	Add 50–100% to the usual treatment amount

Consider the examples in Figs. 2.2 and 2.3.

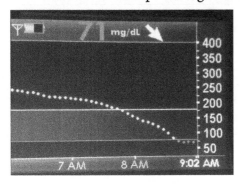

Figure 2.2—SG below target but leveling off.

Fig. 2.2 shows an SG that is below target but leveling off. An individual who normally requires 15 g rapid-acting carbohydrate to treat a low should do fine with this amount.

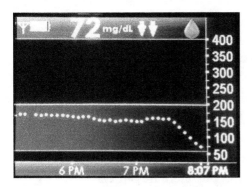

Figure 2.3—SG that is dropping rapidly.

Fig. 2.3 shows an SG that is dropping rapidly. The trend graph and double down arrows both indicate that the glucose will probably continue to drop considerably. An individual who normally requires 15 g rapid-acting carbohydrate should be encouraged to have at least 20–25 g to recover from this low.

Bolus Adjustment

Something that our clinical team has found useful for helping our patients achieve better glycemic control is to teach adjustment of rapid-acting insulin doses (via pump or injection) based on the direction the SG is headed. Why? Consider the purpose of bolus insulin: to have the glucose level back within one's target range by the time the bolus has finished working (typically 3–4 h later). Countless factors are influencing glucose levels at any given time, including active insulin, digesting food, insulin sensitivity, caloric expenditure, and so on. When calculating a bolus, insulin users are usually instructed to consider the current glucose level, the amount of carbohydrate being consumed, and (perhaps) anticipated physical activity. Assuming that the dosing formulas are configured correctly, the calculated dose should work most of the time, right?

Remember, the usual dosing formulas assume that the BG is stable at the time the bolus is given. What if the glucose is rising? Then the BG is likely to be above target when the bolus has finished working. And if the BG is dropping at the time the bolus is given, it is likely to wind up below target.

The presence of up- and down-trend arrows allows us to predict the magnitude and direction of change over the next 30–60 min. Based on our experience, a modest upward or downward trend typically produces a change of at least 25–30 points [1.4–1.7], while a sharp upward or downward trend typically produces a change of at least 50–60 points [2.8–3.3]. So to give yourself (or your patients) the best chance of achieving an in-target glucose over the next several hours, *consider adjusting bolus doses based on the rate of change taking place at the time the bolus is given* (Table 2.4).

Table 2.4—Adjusting Bolus Doses

Current trend	CGM arrow designation	Potential bolus adjustment
Rising modestly	Medtronic: ↑ Dexcom: ↗, ↑	Add enough to usual bolus to offset 25 mg/dL [1.4 mmol/L] rise
Rising sharply	Medtronic: ↑↑ Dexcom: ↑↑	Add enough to usual bolus to offset 50 mg/dL [2.8 mmol/L] rise
Falling modestly	Medtronic: ↓ Dexcom: ↘, ↓	Subtract enough from usual bolus to offset 25 mg/dL [1.4 mmol/L] fall
Falling sharply	Medtronic: ↓↓ Dexcom: ↓↓	Subtract enough from usual bolus to offset 50 mg/dL [2.8 mmol/L] fall

The amount of the bolus adjustment depends on each person's sensitivity to insulin. For someone whose insulin sensitivity (correction factor) is 50 mg/dL [2.8 mmol/L] per unit of insulin, a modest downward trend could be offset with a half-unit reduction in the usual bolus amount. For someone whose sensitivity is 20 mg/dL [1.1 mmol/L] per unit, a sharp rise could be offset with a bolus increase of 2.5 units.

Note that adjusting the bolus by a fixed number of units is more practical than making a percentage adjustment, because we are attempting to offset a specific anticipated rise or fall in the glucose level. Percentage adjustments can vary considerably based on the magnitude of the bolus. For instance, if we were to raise a bolus by 20% for a sharp rise, the increase would be 0.2 units for a 1-unit bolus, and 3 units for a 15-unit bolus. It is sensible to make percentage adjustments when insulin *sensitivity* has been altered due to, say, exercise or illness. But in this instance, we have found a set increase or decrease to be safer and more effective.

Confused yet? Not to worry. The following examples should help.

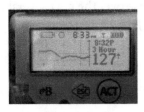

Figure 2.4—Debbie's trend graph.

Debbie is getting ready to bolus for a late dinner (Fig. 2.4). Her fingerstick BG is 145 mg/dL [8.1 mmol/L] and she plans to have 40 g carbohydrate. Her pump calculates a dose of 4.2 units. However, her SG is also rising modestly. She and her physician decided that she should increase her boluses by 0.5 units when the SG is rising modestly and 1 unit when it is rising sharply (her sensitivity or correction factor is 45 mg/dL per unit [2.5 mmol/L per unit]). So she adds 0.5 unit to the 4.2-unit dose suggested by her pump to come up with a total dose of 4.7 units. Taking an extra half-unit increases the likelihood that her SG will be on target a few hours from now.

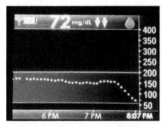

Figure 2.5 — Glen's trend graph.

Glen is having a late dinner, and his trend graph (Fig. 2.5) indicates that his glucose is dropping sharply. Based on the advice of his diabetes educator, Glen not only delays his mealtime insulin but also reduces his usual dose by 2 units (his sensitivity or correction factor is 25 mg/dL [1.4 mmol/L]). Based on his carbs and current fingerstick BG, he calculates an insulin dose of 6.4 units. If he takes his usual 6.4 units, chances are he will wind up below target in the next few hours. By taking 4.4 units, he improves the odds that he will be near his target over the next several hours.

Benefit 3. Reacting to the Alerts

Now, let's consider the real-time use of *high and low alerts*. One of the key benefits of CGM is the ability to detect *approaching* high or low glucose levels. A significant proportion of insulin users suffer from hypoglycemia unawareness[23]—a lack of warning signs to indicate that the glucose level is falling too low. Hypoglycemia unawareness is an adaptive response by the central nervous system to cope more effectively with hypoglycemia. The lack of adrenaline-induced symptoms (e.g., shaking, sweating, rapid heartbeat), however, can allow victims to slip into moderate and severe states of hypoglycemia before the problem is detected and treatment is administered.

I can recall how it felt to have glucose levels drop into the 60s mg/dL [3.5 mmol/L], 70s mg/dL [4.0 mmol/L], or even the 80s mg/dL [4.5 mmol/L] soon after I was diagnosed with type 1 diabetes. The song "Freak Out" was popular at the time, and that's about what it felt like—heart pounding, sweat dripping off my brow, and enough hunger to make wild animals run for cover. As the years progressed, the symptoms mellowed and subsided. BG levels in the 50s mg/dL [3 mmol/L] and 40s mg/dL [2.5 mmol/L] barely caused a jitter. Little did I know that I was a heartbeat away from getting into a car accident, losing consciousness, or worse.

> By acting on alerts in a consistent and constructive manner, the duration and extent of glucose excursions can be minimized.

Research has shown that hypoglycemia unawareness is not limited to people with type 1 diabetes. Those with type 2 diabetes who take insulin or oral hypoglycemic agents experience their share of undetected hypoglycemia as well.[24] In addition to increasing the risk of severe hypoglycemia, hypoglycemia unawareness causes many people to intentionally underdose their insulin[25] and makes intensification of glucose control difficult, if not impossible, from a clinician's standpoint.[26]

Even when hypoglycemia awareness is intact, very few people can tell when their BG is slightly above target or approaching a hypoglycemic range. Although *extreme* highs and lows usually can be felt, modest highs and lows typically go undetected and hence untreated. This, in turn, leads to longer and more extreme glucose excursions.

CGMs provide a warning for mild hypo- and hyperglycemia earlier than most people with diabetes can detect these on their own. Use of rate-of-change alerts and predictive alerts provides an even earlier warning. By acting on alerts in a consistent and constructive manner, the duration and extent of glucose excursions can be minimized.

For example, a sensor that catches an elevated glucose at 200 mg/dL [11.1 mmol/L] allows a user to take corrective action. Rather than waiting for symptoms to appear, the CGM user can act on the high alert by exercising, hydrating, or administering a correction dose of insulin (taking insulin-on-board [IOB] into account). Both the time spent in an above-target range and the magnitude of the high glucose are therefore reduced.

Likewise, a CGM user who is alerted of a falling glucose at 75 mg/dL [4.2 mmol/L] can consume rapidly digesting carbohydrate to minimize a further fall. An individual who relies on the appearance of hypoglycemic symptoms or periodic fingerstick readings may wind up with a significantly lower glucose before treatment begins. Thus, the magnitude of the low and the time spent in a low range can be reduced through early sensor-triggered intervention.

Reducing the amount of time spent in a hypoglycemic range should be of particular interest to those trying to avoid severe hypoglycemia. Research has shown that progression from mild or moderate to severe hypoglycemia has more to do with the length of time spent in a hypoglycemic range than how low the glucose level becomes.[27] Even in the early days of CGM technology, when system performance paled in comparison with what is available today, use of low glucose alerts allowed for early recognition and treatment of hypoglycemia and dramatically reduced the time spent in a hypoglycemic state.[28,29] And, as an added bonus, prevention or avoidance of hypoglycemia is an effective way to restore early warning signs and normal counter-regulatory responses.[30]

Low alerts can make it safer for anyone at risk of hypoglycemia (insulin, sulfonylurea, or meglitinide users) to work, drive, exercise, sleep, and aim for tighter glycemic control. Likewise, the high alerts allow more aggressive management of after-meal glucose spikes, prevention of ketoacidosis, and lowering of the HbA_{1c}. Of course, this hinges on CGM system performance and appropriate calibration. And for the alerts to be beneficial to the user, appropriate alert settings and timely responses are essential.

High and Low Alerts

High- and low-alert levels are not the same as a person's target glucose range. For example, if someone is content keeping their glucose between 70 and 160 mg/dL [3.9 and 8.9 mmol/L], setting the low alert at 70 mg/dL [3.9 mmol/L] would not be an effective way to keep the glucose from dropping to <70 mg/dL [3.9 mmol/L]. Why? First, there is the matter of lag time. When glucose levels are falling, the sensor value will typically be higher than the BG. An SG value of 70 mg/dL [3.9 mmol/L] will often correspond with a BG value in the 50s or 60s mg/dL [3–3.5 mmol/L]. The faster the glucose is falling, such as during exercise, the greater the discrepancy. Second, if you want to prevent hypoglycemia, you can't wait until you're already low (Fig. 2.6).

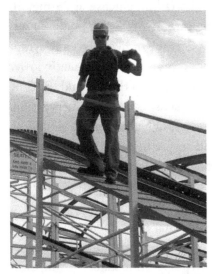

Figure 2.6—Jon Mahony, amusement park technician, counts on his CGM to keep himself safe while he works at great heights to make sure the rides are safe.

Logic and experience dictate that setting the low alert *above* the hypoglycemia threshold (low point of one's target range) is necessary to prevent lows. As a general guideline, consider setting your low threshold 10–20 mg/dL [0.6–1.1 mmol/L] points above the lowest reading that you consider acceptable (Table 2.5).

Table 2.5—Low-Alert Settings

If you want to keep your BG above this level (mg/dL [mmol/L])	Set your low alert at this level (mg/dL [mmol/L])
60 [3.3]	70–80 [3.9–4.4]
70 [3.9]	80–90 [4.4–5.0]
80 [4.4]	90–100 [5.0–5.6]
90 [5.0]	100–110 [5.6–6.1]

BG, blood glucose.

Given the inexact nature of SG readings, the higher the low alert is set, the greater the chance for false alerts. Many of our clients have found it helpful to start with a relatively high low-alert threshold and then lower it if false alerts become a nuisance.

Setting the high alerts takes a bit more thought. Most people with diabetes experience far more high than low glucose readings. The danger associated with a single high is much lower than the risk created by a single low (assuming ketones and ketoacidosis are not involved), and so it is important to balance the value of high alerts with the nuisance that they can cause. I have seen countless individuals who literally gave up on CGM because the alerts were occurring far too often. They either started to ignore the alerts or stopped using the system entirely.

When someone is using a CGM for the first time, it is reasonable to either turn off the high alerts or set them at an extremely high level. Once a user becomes comfortable and familiar with the system—typically a couple of weeks after starting—it makes sense to start lowering the high-alert threshold. Keep in mind that the high alert ultimately should correspond with an individual's highest acceptable *post*meal glucose level, not the *pre*meal level. Otherwise, the alerts will occur after virtually every meal and snack.

For example, many people are encouraged to keep their peak postmeal glucose <180 mg/dL [10 mmol/L]. When this is the case, the following high-alert settings may be utilized (Table 2.6).

Table 2.6—Intensification of High-Alert Settings

Time since initiation	High-alert setting (mg/dL [mmol/L])
CGM startup	300 [16.7]
2 weeks	250 [13.9]
1 month	220 [12.2]
2 months	200 [11.2]
3 months	180 [10.0]

CGM, continuous glucose monitoring.

The whole lag-time issue applies to rising as well as falling glucose levels. When levels are rising, we typically observe SG values that are lower than BG values. Those who can tolerate the extra alerts may choose to set the high alert 10–20 mg/dL [0.6–1.1 mmol/L] points *below* the highest acceptable postmeal glucose.

To benefit from alerts, one's response should be timely, appropriate, and consistent. With high alerts, there is a natural tendency to "fix" the problem with extra insulin. Many people neglect to consider active (unused) insulin from a prior dose when doing so, and wind up low as a result. The term *angry/rage bolus* was coined in the diabetes online community to denote this type of behavior.

It is essential to take active mealtime insulin (also called IOB or bolus-on-board) into account when treating above-target glucose values, and deduct it from the usual correction dose. Most insulin pumps do this automatically, but those individuals who take insulin by injection will need to calculate IOB by hand. For simplicity, we created the following chart (based on postcorrection-bolus glucose profiles observed in our clients' CGM reports) to estimate IOB when taking rapid-acting insulin (aspart, lispro, glulisine) by injection (Table 2.7).

> To benefit from alerts, one's response should be timely, appropriate, and consistent.

Table 2.7 — Calculating IOB*

Time since rapid-acting insulin was given	0.5 h	1 h	1.5 h	2 h	2.5 h	3 h	3.5 h	4 h
Insulin "used up"	10%	30%	50%	65%	80%	90%	95%	100%
Insulin still "on board"	90%	70%	50%	35%	20%	10%	5%	0%

*IOB, insulin-on-board.

For example, someone who took 6 units of insulin for a 3 P.M. snack and then checked their glucose at 5 P.M. still has 35% of their bolus remaining (6 units × 35% = 2 units of IOB). Deducting this amount from any correction dose that would have normally been given for the 5 P.M. BG reading would reduce the chances of subsequent hypoglycemia.

As long as ketones are not present, it is also reasonable to respond to high alerts with physical activity that is known to lower the BG. Low-to-moderate-intensity cardiovascular (aerobic) exercise is often a good choice.[31] Whether insulin or physical activity is used to reverse an elevated or rising glucose, it is important to take steps promptly and consistently. This is the best way to minimize the duration and magnitude of above-target glucose levels.

Responding to low alerts is a bit more straightforward. When a low alert occurs, it will almost always be necessary to consume carbohydrates. By definition, the glucose level will be falling when the low threshold is crossed, so the actual BG is likely to be lower than the number displayed on the screen. Per FDA labeling guidelines, a fingerstick is recommended to verify the glucose value and to determine the exact amount of carbs needed. But as a general rule, with every low alert, eat something that will raise the BG quickly. This will minimize the duration and severity of the low, and in some cases, prevent it altogether.

Rate-of-Change Alerts

All CGM systems have the ability to alert users when the glucose level is rising or falling quickly. The fall rate can offer a great deal of utility to those who are trying to avoid hypoglycemia, because adjustments might be necessary even when the glucose is normal or moderately elevated.

Fall-rate alerts occur most often during exercise or the peak action time of rapid-acting insulin. Based on my experience, it is best to set the fall rate at 3 mg/dL/min [0.2 mmol/L/min]. When glucose levels are dropping at this rate over the past 15–20 min, action may be necessary to prevent subsequent hypoglycemia (Table 2.8).

Table 2.8—Suggested Responses to Fall-Rate Alerts

Current glucose	Response with fall alert
Normal range	Consume rapid-acting carbs
Slightly above normal	Check again in 15–20 min
Well above normal	Check again in 30–60 min

The practical value of rise-rate alerts is questionable. These alerts typically occur after food consumption, particularly when consuming rapidly digesting (high-glycemic-index) forms of carbohydrate. In many cases, frequent rise-rate alerts lead to "alert fatigue" and a tendency for the user to ignore alerts completely.

Another challenge with using rise alerts is how to respond to them, because they often take place when a great deal of mealtime insulin is still working. Rise alerts that occur at other times of day may indicate problems, such as the following:

- Compromised infusion from an insulin pump
- Forgetting to bolus for an earlier meal or snack
- Spoiled insulin
- A missed dose of diabetes medication
- An adverse reaction to a medication
- A stress response

◆ An intense allergic reaction
◆ Developing illness or infection

In these instances, appropriate troubleshooting, including ketone testing and communication with one's health-care team, can prevent prolonged hyperglycemia or ketoacidosis. For those who choose to use rise alerts, a setting of 3.0 mg/dL/min [0.2 mmol/L/min] is suggested.

Predictive Alerts

Predictive alerts are analogous to weather forecasts, particularly in locations where the weather varies from day to day. Weather forecasts are based on historical evidence, scientific models, and the interpretive skills of the forecaster. In most cases, forecasters can predict tomorrow's weather pretty accurately. The three-day forecast is a bit less precise, and the seven-day forecast is usually little more than a shot in the dark.

BG levels follow patterns that are at times predictable and at times seemingly random. Predictive alerts are based on the current glucose level and the recent upward or downward trend. These alerts *assume* that the current trend will continue without wavering. Falling glucose will continue to fall at its current rate, and rising glucose will continue to rise at its current rate. The fact is, sometimes they do, but more often than not, their course (like that of a hurricane) deviates from what the models predict. The further out you try to predict, the less accurate the prediction becomes.

Low predictive alerts have inherent value for those trying to avoid hypoglycemia. To minimize the incidence of false positive alerts (predicted lows that never actually become lows), set the time duration for the prediction as short as possible. It is a lot easier to accurately predict what will happen in the next 5 to 10 min than it is to predict what will happen in 15 to 20 min.

Responses to predictive low alerts mirror those of fall-rate alerts. Consumption of rapid-acting carbohydrate is recommended for the prevention of subsequent hypoglycemia, although slightly less carbohydrate may be needed compared with that required for treating a glucose level that is already in a hypoglycemic range. A diabetes educator can help devise an individualized plan to address predictive low alerts.

Clinically, I have found that high predictive alerts tend to offer very little value to users. Their accuracy is generally poor due to the fact that previous mealtime insulin can change the course of a rising trend very quickly, resulting in frustration on the part of users. My suggestion is to keep the predictive high alerts turned off.

Benefit 4. Pump Automation

Another way CGM can be of use in real time is through integration with an insulin delivery device and automation of insulin delivery. Several insulin pump and CGM manufacturers are working toward a system that ultimately will keep glucose levels within a normal range around the clock. Such a system, commonly referred to as an "artificial pancreas" or "closed loop," is still in development. For now, though, CGM users can benefit from small (but significant) steps that are being taken toward a fully automated system.

As of the publication of this book, only the Medtronic sensor and Medtronic pump have achieved any level of integration and automation, although a number of other device companies are reported to be close to releasing their own versions. The Medtronic Veo or 530G system offers a *low shut-off* (also called *threshold suspend*) feature, whereby basal insulin delivery is halted automatically for up to 2 h whenever the SG falls below the low threshold set by the user. Use of this feature is optional and should be individualized based on the needs of the user.

The advantage of the low shut-off feature should be obvious: In the event of a hypoglycemic episode that renders the victim unable to self-treat (or ask for help), halting the basal insulin should cause the glucose to eventually rise on its own. Medtronic's research has shown that use of the threshold suspend feature reduces the length of time spent in a hypoglycemic range without producing significant hyperglycemia after the fact.[32] As noted previously, lows that continue for many hours put a person at risk of severe hypoglycemia (seizure, continued loss of consciousness, coma). By limiting the time spent in a hypoglycemic state, the low suspend feature can help to keep a moderate low from becoming more severe.

Earlier, we discussed the prevalence and safety risks associated with hypoglycemia unawareness. Even those with good hypoglycemia recognition are susceptible to problems at night. Hypoglycemic episodes that occur during sleep may not cause a person to wake on his or her own. Research on Medtronic's low shut-off feature showed a 30% reduction in the incidence of nighttime hypoglycemia without any increase in HbA_{1c} when the feature is utilized.[26]

Likewise, hypoglycemia that is accompanied by alcohol consumption or an accident may keep a victim from seeking or receiving proper treatment. In situations like these, the automated low shut-off feature may help to keep a minor problem from becoming a major one. Low shut-off thus serves as an emergency last-resort method for escaping severe hypoglycemia when no other treatment is available or possible. This, in turn, can provide emotional comfort to loved ones and caregivers.

So why wouldn't everyone use the low shut-off feature? There are a few reasons. First, suspending basal insulin is not the best way to treat everyday, garden-variety bouts of hypoglycemia. Consumption of rapid-acting carbohydrate typically will raise the glucose within 15–30 min, whereas basal suspension typically takes 1–2 h or more.[33] Notably, the low shut-off is activated *by default* whenever the SG falls below the low threshold. If the user eats to treat the low and does not remember to reactivate basal delivery, they are essentially double-treating the low, and an undesired high glucose may result. In addition, there is the ever-present chance of experiencing false positives—low alerts (and basal suspensions) that occur when the glucose is not actually low.

In deciding whether to use the low shut-off feature, one must weigh the potential benefits against the potential drawbacks. For those who spend a great deal of time alone, have hypoglycemia unawareness, and are susceptible to severe lows, the scale is tilted heavily toward use of the feature. For those with good hypoglycemia recognition, adequate social support, or a desire to minimize the frequency of alerts, the scale tends to tilt the other way. As CGM accuracy continues to improve and pump-sensor integration advances to the point at which lows (and highs) can be *prevented*, use of automated pump-sensor features will no doubt become more universal.

CHAPTER 3

Improving Control with CGM Data Analysis

Evaluation of the DCCT patients followed at the International Dia-
betes Center showed that one of the five identified factors associated
with a lower HbA$_{1c}$ was... whether individuals actually reviewed
their glucose records and made self-adjustments based on principles
including pattern management.

—Pearson and Bergenstal[34]

The statement by Pearson and Bergenstal says a lot. This chapter is all about making things better by learning from history. Whether you're a person with diabetes trying not to make the same mistakes twice or a health-care provider looking to offer up a few pearls of wisdom to your patients, CGMs provide a wealth of valuable downloadable information. Retrospective analysis of that information is one of the keys to benefiting from CGM use.[35]

ABOUT THE SOFTWARE

A number of software programs allow CGM users and their clinicians to obtain key statistics and view CGM data in a graphic and customized format. Without downloading, the user (and their clinician) typically can access only the most recent 24 h of data on the receiver screen. And because diabetes subscribes to the philosophy that "on any given day, anything can happen," it is simply not practical to make therapy adjustments based on a single day's data or a single incident.

Effective therapy adjustments are derived through *pattern analysis*—detection of events that repeat on a regular or semiregular basis. Pattern analysis is what allows us to play diabetes detective: figuring out the causes of and solutions to those patterns.

> Effective therapy adjustments are derived through *pattern analysis*— detection of events that repeat on a regular or semiregular basis.

The purpose of CGM download software is to present data in a meaningful way. There is a gradual movement toward offering guided assistance with the analysis of the data as well. Table 3.1 provides a summary of currently available software programs.

Table 3.1—Software Programs

CGM system	Download program	Useful reports	Compatibility and use
Dexcom	Dexcom Studio	• Patterns • Daily Trends • Glucose Trend • Success Report	PC only; data file sharable via e-mail
	Diasend	• Modal (CGM tab) • Day-by-Day (CGM tab) • Compilation	Web based; Mac or PC compatible; requires "uploader" software on computer; easily shared data
Medtronic	CareLink	• Sensor Daily Overlay • Sensor Overlay by Meal • Daily Summary • Trends Summary	Web based; PC and Mac compatible; data/reports easily sharable (password required)
	CareLink Pro	• Therapy Management Dashboard • Episode Summary • Adherence	PC only; intended for health care provider use

CGM, continuous glucose monitoring.

Dexcom Studio software (go to www.dexcom.com to install) is designed exclusively for downloading and displaying data from Dexcom receivers. It is PC based and not web enabled, and it does not currently work on Mac systems. Users who would like to share their data with a health-care provider may do so by saving their "patient file" and sending it as an e-mail attachment (the recipient would then load the patient's file using the Studio software on their computer). This is accomplished by doing the following:

1. Click on the "Patients" tab.
2. Highlight the appropriate name.
3. Select "Save Patient File."
4. Save the file to a place where you can easily find it on your computer; you may change the name of the file, but do not change the extension (it must be .patient).
5. Attach this file to an e-mail.

On the recipient or health-care provider's side, the procedure is as follows:

1. Save the e-mail attachment to your computer (I have a folder dedicated to these types of files); do not change the file extension (it must be .patient).
2. Open Studio software.
3. Click on the "Patients" tab.
4. Select "Load Patient File."
5. Click on the patient that you just loaded and then view their reports; in some cases, the patient's name does not appear in the list, so if you have multiple patients in your database, you may need to search by the device serial number (usually part of the saved file name) or the date of the last upload.

It is usually necessary to customize the target glucose range before generating reports. This option can be found at the top of most of the report screens. Studio integrates seamlessly with Microsoft Word to quickly print reports that are displayed on screen.

The Patterns report in Studio produces a one-page data summary that includes statistical information and a standard day (24-h) graph with multiple days superimposed for pattern analysis. The Daily Trends report also produces a standard day graph, but also gives the option of sorting data by glucose range(s), time(s) of day, and day(s) of the week. Below the Daily Trends graph is a detailed statistical summary broken down by hour of the day. Because very few people adhere to the same meal, snack, sleep, work, and exercise schedule every day, the value of this data is somewhat limited. Similarly, the Hourly Stats report, which shows averages, standard deviations, and glucose ranges broken down by hour, will be difficult to interpret unless the user's schedule is the same from day to day. The Glucose Trend report provides a look at sensor data for individual days and includes details from any event markers (insulin, food, exercise) that were entered by the user. The Success Report offers an opportunity to see how SG statistics have changed over time. Data can be compared from one week to the next, one month to the next, or one quarter to the next, which is an excellent way to evaluate therapy changes that were made recently.

The independent web-based program Diasend (go to www.diasend.com to register and download the uploader software) imports and merges data from a variety of devices (including BG meters, insulin pumps, and the Dexcom CGM). It can be used on just about any computer that has Internet access. An "uploader" software must be installed on the user's (or clinician's) computer to transmit data to the website. Health-care providers (clinics) have the opportunity to set up accounts on Diasend so that patients can share their data automatically when they download. Users have the option of entering their clinic's identification number during registration so that their reports are accessible to their health-care provider. Otherwise, patients can share their login details with their clinician so that reports can be viewed at the clinician's office.

Once data have been downloaded, the "CGM" tab in Diasend serves as a portal to several useful reports. The default graph that appears is similar to the Daily Trends graph in Dexcom's Studio software, and has limited value unless the user keeps a consistent schedule from day to day. Clicking on "Box/Plot Modal" produces daily SG tracings superimposed for trend analysis purposes. Day-by-Day reports provide a series of single-day Glucose Trend Graphs with notations for calibration values, as well as carbohydrate entries and insulin delivery (if a pump was also downloaded). The "Compilation" tab provides statistical reports for CGM data, along with BG, insulin, and carb data if a pump or meter was also downloaded.

Medtronic offers two programs for downloading data from their real-time and professional-use CGM systems: CareLink Personal and CareLink Pro. CareLink Personal is web based and accessible through both PC and Mac computers (go to https://carelink.minimed.com to access). No software needs to be installed, but a transmission device (CareLink USB or Contour Next Link USB meter) must be used to transmit data from the pump through the computer and to the website. These devices can be obtained from Medtronic. Once downloaded, reports can be accessed by the user and their health-care providers by entering a username and passcode. Users should take the time to set their typical mealtimes and target glucose ranges in the "Preferences" tab before generating reports and analyzing data.

Several useful reports are available in CareLink Personal. The Sensor Daily Overlay report yields a 24-h tracing, with up to 7 days superimposed for trend analysis purposes. Daily and weekly statistics are generated, along with accuracy data (comparing sensor and calibration values) for the days being evaluated. When a sensor-augmented Medtronic insulin pump is downloaded, the Sensor Overlay by Meal provides a unique look at up to 7 days of postmeal sensor tracings. The system detects the time that a meal bolus was delivered and marks this as the "start" time. The sensor tracing for the following 4 h is displayed, with up to 7 days superimposed. Breakfast, lunch, and dinner time intervals are displayed separately. This report is excellent for determining the magnitude of postmeal glucose peaks as well as the effectiveness of the mealtime dose. CareLink Personal can generate detailed single-day Daily Summary reports. These reports provide SG and BG data at the top of the report, basal and bolus insulin delivery (with temp basals and suspensions noted) in the middle, and carbohydrate entries and physical activity (entered manually) at the bottom. Another helpful report for those using a sensor-augmented insulin pump is the Trends Summary. Although sensor data do not appear on this report, it provides a statistical summary of fingerstick BG data, insulin use, and carbohydrate intake over a specified time interval. Because many reports are usually desired when using Carelink Personal, I recommend using the batch reporting feature. Multiple reports (with variable date ranges, if desired) can be selected and generated simultaneously.

CareLink Pro is a PC-based software program that allows health-care professionals to see more details than are available in CareLink Personal. The Pro software also detects patterns that can guide clinicians in coming to therapeutic conclusions. CareLink Pro *can* also be used by patients if a copy of the software (on CD only) is provided by the clinician. Medtronic representatives can provide extra copies of the software at their discretion. Once the software is installed on a computer, data must be imported from CareLink Personal, so each patient's device must be downloaded to CareLink Personal first.

Although CareLink Pro reports can appear complex, valuable and unique insights can be derived. For example, the Adherence report indicates the frequency of insulin pump infusion site changes and cannula fills, time spent in a state of pump suspension, and situations in which the pump user has delivered a bolus dose that differs from what the pump's bolus calculator (Bolus Wizard) recommended. The Dashboard report specifies times of day when patterns of hypoglycemia and hyperglycemia are most common and provides an expanded view of SG values around mealtimes (from 1 h premeal to 5 h postmeal) superimposed for postprandial trend analysis. The type and frequency of sensor alerts are also included in this report.

The Episode Summary report is what puts the "pro" in CareLink Pro. This report totals the number of high and low alerts within a chosen date range and categories the events that *preceded* the alerts so that cause-and-effect relationships may be established. For example, the report may indicate that 10 low-glucose alerts occurred in the past month, and 9 of the 10 alerts were preceded by correction boluses for high glucose. Or, it may indicate that 50% of high alerts occurred when an infusion set was used for longer than usual. Although there is no way to prove that the preceding events are the direct cause of glucose control issues, the reports provide a good starting point for investigation and problem solving.

From a clinical standpoint, one can debate the benefit and value of CareLink Pro versus CareLink Personal. Personally, I find CareLink Personal reports to be clear, concise, and detailed enough to form intelligent conclusions. When glucose control issues run rampant and I find myself searching for more answers, CareLink Pro reports can provide additional insights.

Qualification Counts

Before evaluating a set of CGM data, it is important to *qualify* the information. This means verifying that the data ARE reliable and representative of the user's true patterns. Take a moment to answer the following four questions before diving into the data:

1. *Are the clock and date set correctly on the receiver?* An A.M./P.M. reversal can lead to a complete misunderstanding of what actually took place.
2. *Were sufficient calibrations performed?* A system that was undercalibrated may lead the analyzer on a "wild glucose chase."

3. *What were the conditions under which the data were collected?* Do they represent a typical situation, or were there extenuating circumstances, such as unusual stress, travel, activity, illness, or use of steroid medications?

4. *Were the data reasonably accurate?* Although some inaccuracy is expected, gross inaccuracy can cause us to draw incorrect conclusions. In the Medtronic system, take a look at the mean absolute difference (MAD) percentage for the full week on the Sensor Daily Overlay report. If the MAD is >15–18% for the time period being evaluated, the data may not be worth reviewing. On the Dexcom Daily Trend reports, observe the discrepancy between the calibration values (denoted as red diamonds) and the simultaneous SG values (the blue dots). If there are consistent large discrepancies, consider passing up on the data analysis (see the example in Fig. 3.1).

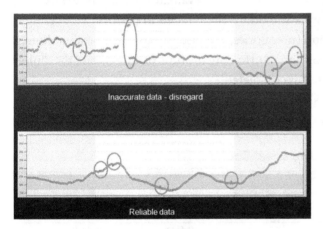

Figure 3.1 — Inaccurate versus reliable data.

It's in the Preparation

Every good house painter knows that proper preparation of the work surface is the key to success. The same can be said for analyzing CGM data. Looking at a bunch of numbers, charts, and graphs of glucose values will only get you so far. If you really want to learn something, it is important to know the *context* in which the data were collected.

When using a *professional CGM* (a system worn temporarily for analysis purposes), it helps to have details to go along with the SG reports. The CGM user should keep a written or computerized log* of the following:

- Timing and content of meals
- Duration and nature of exercise
- Doses of insulin and other diabetes medications
- Noteworthy events (e.g., restaurant meals, illnesses, unusual stress, pump infusion set changes, menses)

> It is important to know the *context* of the glucose data.

For those who prefer an electronic form of logging, some professional CGMs allow the user to input event markers that will appear in specific downloaded reports. Use the event markers consistently unless written logging is performed.

In addition, for CGM users who take basal insulin by injection, a professional CGM session is a *golden* opportunity to evaluate the dose. While wearing the professional CGM, users should be encouraged to perform an overnight fast on at least one occasion (no calories, exercise, or rapid insulin after dinner, until breakfast the next morning) and to note the time of dinner (and the dinner bolus) on the nights this test is completed.

Insulin pump users should be encouraged to perform a series of fasts at various times of day to evaluate the pump's basal settings (Table 3.2).

Table 3.2—Tests to Evaluate Basal Settings

Basal test	Eat and bolus by	Then no calories, boluses, or exercise until	Evaluate sensor data between
Overnight	6 p.m.	7 a.m.	10 p.m. and 7 a.m.
Morning	11 p.m.	12 noon (skip breakfast)	7 a.m. and 12 noon
Afternoon	8 a.m.	5 p.m. (skip lunch)	12 noon and 5 p.m.
Evening	1 p.m.	10 p.m. (late dinner)	5 p.m. and 10 p.m.

It is best to have a healthy, low-fat (non-restaurant) meal before the test to prevent extended digestion, along with a normal (non-extended) bolus of insulin. No *calories* may be consumed during a basal test, as even small amounts of protein and fat, in the absence of carbohydrate, can influence glucose levels.[36] The test should be canceled if hypoglycemia occurs or the

---

*Free logsheets can be found on my website: integrateddiabetes.com/diabetic-logsheets. The sheets may be printed and reproduced, or saved on one's computer for typing the data directly onto the form.

glucose rises and remains well above target several hours after the meal. Details about evaluating the sensor data during basal tests will be covered later in this chapter.

Similarly, those using a *personal CGM* system can learn 10 times more, and help their health-care professional in the process, by keeping detailed notes or using the CGM's event markers. In most cases, recording key data (insulin doses, meals/snacks, exercise) for 1 or 2 weeks provides sufficient data for performing an effective analysis of CGM data.

Fun with Statistics

Unlike fingerstick BG meters, CGMs collect data around the clock: before meals, between meals, after meals, and while we sleep, exercise, fantasize, and procrastinate. When functioning properly and worn consistently, CGMs generate hundreds of SG values per day. The data are not skewed by checking multiple times during highs or lows or by checking only before eating. They are a true reflection of day-to-day around-the-clock glucose levels. As such, the statistics generated by CGMs are of much greater value than the statistics garnered from downloading BG meters.

The *mean (average)* SG represents a fairly true average, albeit slightly lower than reality because of a natural tendency for the systems to err on the side of lower rather than higher values, and the prolonged lag time that occurs when recovering from hypoglycemia. Adding 2–3% to an SG average is a good way to correct for these system inadequacies. In fact, I have found it fairly easy to estimate an A1C based on 1–3 months of sensor data:

1. Take the average glucose for the past 1, 2, or 3 months from the CGM download.
2. Multiply the average by 1.03 (to correct for system error).
3. To this "true average," add 46.7, and then divide by 28.7. If measuring in molar solutions (i.e., mmol/L), take the result from step 2, add 2.59, and divide by 1.59. This is called an "estimated average glucose" equation based on A1C.[37]

Another useful statistic is the *standard deviation*. This represents the amount of variability in the glucose levels. Technically, if you add and subtract the standard deviation from the mean (average), you get a range that includes 68% of the glucose values. For example, with an average of 180 mg/dL [10 mmol/L] and a standard deviation of 72 mg/dL [4 mmol/L], 68% of the readings are between 108 and 252 mg/dL [6 and 14 mmol/L]. A high standard deviation means that there are a lot of values that are way above or below the average—a lot of bouncing around, so to speak. A low standard deviation indicates that the glucose levels have been relatively stable.

Why is it important to look at the amount of variance? For starters, anyone who tracks their glucose closely knows that rapid and significant swings tend to affect one's performance on a daily basis. Rapid rises can cause tiredness, difficulty concentrating, impaired physical performance, and mood changes.[38] Rapid falls can cause hypoglycemia-type sensations without actually being low. In addition, a growing body of research is indicating that variability in glucose, and not just the overall average (as reflected by A1C), affects one's risk for developing long-term diabetes complications.[39-41]

In general, a standard deviation that is <33% (one-third) of the average is desirable. A standard deviation that is >50% (half) of the average indicates too much time spent in extreme high and low glucose zones.

Speaking of zones, another very useful statistic is the amount of time spent above, below, and within one's target glucose range. The target range can be customized on each software program, and should be individualized for each person. And remember, target ranges should *not* be the same as the high- and low-alert thresholds.

Current American Diabetes Association Standards of Care call for premeal capillary glucose (fingerstick) for nonpregnant adults to fall between 80 and 130 mg/dL [4.4 and 7.2 mmol/L], with a peak postprandial glucose of <180 mg/dL [10 mmol/L].[22] It is strongly recommended, however, that individualization be based on each person's goals, capabilities, and risk factors. Slightly higher glucose targets are suggested for both children and the elderly (90–130 mg/dL [5.0–7.2 mmol/L] premeal, 90–150 mg/dL [5.0–8.3 mmol/L] at bedtime and overnight). Lower targets are recommended for gestational diabetes (≤95 mg/dL [5.3 mmol/L] premeal, ≤140 mg/dL [7.8 mmol/L] 1 h postmeal, ≤120 mg/dL [6.7 mmol/L] 2 h postmeal), and pregnancy with preexisting diabetes (60–99 mg/dL [3.3–5.4 mmol/L] premeal, 100–129 mg/dL [5.4–7.1 mmol/L] postmeal).[42]

For most of the patients in my practice, customized and realistic target ranges appear as shown in Table 3.3.

Table 3.3—Customized and Realistic Target Ranges

Overall target (mg/dL)	Overall target (mmol/L)	Population
70–120	4–7	• Type 2 diabetes, not taking mealtime insulin
60–140	3.5–8	• Type 1 diabetes during pregnancy • Gestational diabetes
70–160	4–9	• Most intensive insulin users • Reasonable hypoglycemia awareness (or using CGM)
80–180	4.5–10	• Insulin users with history of severe hypoglycemia or hypoglycemia unawareness • Heart disease
80–200	4.5–11	• Very young children • Adolescents with poor control • Elderly

Some software, such as CareLink, allows the use of different target ranges in pre- and postmeal time intervals. When this is the case, we usually set the postmeal ranges ~25% higher than the premeal ranges. For example, if the premeal target is 70–160 mg/dL [4–9 mmol/L], the postmeal range would be ~90–200 mg/dL [5–11 mmol/L].

One of our major goals is to spend as much time within the target range as possible, and as little time above and below target. It is reasonable for most people to attain ≥70% time within range, but this may take time and work to achieve. It may be more of a challenge for young children, adolescents, and those with very erratic schedules. What is really important is to make steady progress toward a desired goal.

The percent of time spent *below* the target range is of particular importance to everyone with diabetes, particularly those with hypoglycemia unawareness or a history of severe hypoglycemia. In most cases, we recommend spending <5% of one's time below target. Although 5% may not seem like much, it represents an average of 1 h and 12 min in a hypoglycemic range each day.

Although numeric data can be used to evaluate the percent of time spent above, below, and within one's target range, I am partial to looking at pie charts for a quick visual assessment of one's progress and performance (Fig. 3.2).

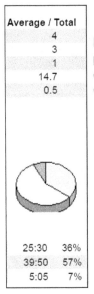

Average / Total
4
3
1
14.7
0.5

25:30	36%
39:50	57%
5:05	7%

Figure 3.2—Visual assessment of progress and performance. Up to a 1-week sensor statistical summary can be found on the far-right side of the Sensor Daily Overlay report on CareLink Personal.

Statistics	
Glucose Average	148 mg/dL
Sensor Usage	10 of 14 Days
Calibrations / day	2.1
Standard Deviation	± 41 mg/dL
	32 % High
	65 % Target
	2 % Low
Target Range	80 - 160 mg/dL
Nighttime Range	10:00 PM - 6:00 AM

Figure 3.3—Sensor statistical summary. The statistical summary from a Dexcom Studio's Patterns report provides a quick look at time spent above, below, and within target range.

Finally, it may be useful to quantify the number of times the glucose has gone above or below alert thresholds within a given time interval (such as a week or a month). Medtronic's CareLink Professional software does this automatically in its Episode Summary report. It is fairly easy to count the episodes on a standard day report in the other programs. Setting short-term goals to reduce the number of high and low episodes can be an effective motivator for applying new glucose management strategies.

TURNING SPAGHETTI INTO INSIGHT

Have you ever stared really closely at a 7- to 14-day CGM modal-day trend graph or pattern report? Some view it as a tangled mass of multicolored spaghetti. It sort of makes one's eyes cross. Trying to analyze these types of reports without a solid game plan is a good way to become confused and frustrated. Rather than going into the graphic reports with an open mind, *set yourself up with a solid agenda.*

You can derive a number of important conclusions (I call them "brilliant insights") from the trend graphs. These include the following:

◆ Uncovering patterns of hypoglycemia
◆ Seeking the dark side of the moon (evaluating what's going on *between* fingersticks)
◆ Measuring the magnitude of postprandial (after-meal) glucose spikes
◆ Determining the effectiveness of mealtime insulin doses
◆ Quantifying the correction factor–insulin sensitivity
◆ Verifying that basal insulin levels are set properly
◆ Learning the duration of the insulin action curve
◆ Evaluating the treatment of hypoglycemia
◆ Titrating incretin medications
◆ Discovering the impact of lifestyle events and activities
◆ Revealing system abuses or behaviors that may be sabotaging one's control

Now let's take a look at some examples.

Brilliant Insight 1.
Uncovering Patterns of Hypoglycemia

There's an unwritten rule in the diabetes world: Fix the lows first. Besides serving as an imminent danger, hypoglycemia often causes hormonal changes that can wreak havoc on glucose control for several hours. In many cases, fixing the lows will also fix subsequent highs. Thus, we start by looking for patterns of hypoglycemia.

Reviewing a batch of daily sensor graphs allows us to see whether hypo-glycemia is taking place at specific times of day. Despite the fact that fingerstick readings are recommended to confirm hypoglycemia, the reality is that many people simply treat their symptoms without actually testing, so patterns of lows may not show up in a meter download. For CGM users, it is possible that the pattern was not noticed when it was buried in a muddle of daily activities and fluctuations. Or perhaps the lows took place at a time when the CGM user was oblivious to his or her own symptoms and the sensor alerts (assuming the alerts were activated). That's why we look at the graphs.

Case Study 3.1: Melissa

Most of the college students that I work with prefer to communicate via quick snippets of information: data downloads, e-mails, text messages, and so on. When Melissa, a student at Columbia University, e-mailed me that she was seeing unusual rises in her morning glucose without eating breakfast, our natural instinct would be to raise her basal insulin in the morning. However, her sensor data looked like this (Fig. 3.4):

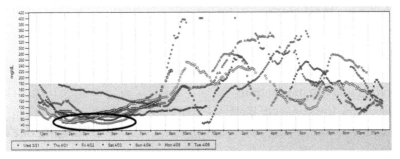

Figure 3.4—Melissa's sensor data.

Observation: Melissa's report is confirmed. Her glucose is indeed rising in the morning. But notice that she is experiencing mild hypoglycemia just about every night between 2 A.M. and 6 A.M.

Conclusion: Clearly, the morning rises are the result of the undetected and untreated lows in the middle of the night (Dr. Somogyi would be proud of our little discovery). The sudden appearance of lows in the middle of the night begs the question: What is causing them? I asked Melissa about her nighttime snack/bolus, exercise, and drinking patterns. As it turns out, she recently joined a sorority and was drinking in the evening on a regular basis. We discussed the delayed effects of alcohol on glucose levels. Melissa opted to cut back on weekday drinking and to use temporary basal reductions on her pump when she drinks on weekends.

Brilliant Insight 2.
Seeking the Dark Side of the Moon*

Fingerstick data, whether downloaded, written down, or observed by scrolling through the meter's memory, miss a great deal. Someone who checks their BG four times daily goes an average of 6 h between readings. That's 6 h with no idea what their glucose level actually is. Someone who checks twice daily spends an average of 12 h in the dark.

Although CGM has potential benefit for those with type 1 diabetes who monitor their BG frequently, it also can be useful for those with type 2 diabetes who are not on an intensive insulin program and may not be checking glucose levels all that often. Of course, it is still necessary to perform sufficient fingersticks to calibrate the CGM properly.

Continuous sensor data can help explain discrepancies between self-monitoring results and lab values, and may serve as a valuable guide in knowing when one's therapy needs to be changed or intensified. Of course, real-time CGM provides an opportunity to immediately discover how one's daily food and activity choices influence glucose control.

Case Study 3.2: Esther

The Dexcom Studio Daily Trends report below was taken from Esther—a woman with type 2 diabetes who takes oral agents only (metformin and sitagliptin). She checks her glucose once daily (first thing in the morning), and the readings are almost always in a normal range, but her last A1C was 8%. She agreed to step her fingerstick checks up to twice daily to calibrate her CGM in the morning and evening (Fig. 3.5).

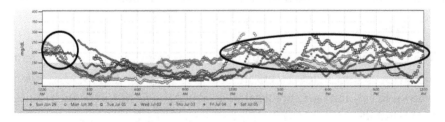

Figure 3.5—Esther's Daily Trends report.

---

*My apologies to Pink Floyd.

Observation: What Esther's *fasting* glucose readings didn't tell us is that she is spending most of the remainder of the day above her target range, with a significant rise starting after lunch. What appear to be mild lows in the middle of the night and morning are, in all likelihood, slight sensor inaccuracies because Esther's treatment plan does not include a hypoglycemia-inducing agent.

Conclusion: Esther may be having too much carbohydrate at lunch or dinner, or she could be snacking heavily in the afternoon and evening. She would benefit from a review of her meal plan and education on proper distribution of carbohydrates throughout the day. It is also possible that her current medication doses are insufficient or that she requires an addition to her medical therapy.

Brilliant Insight 3.
Measuring the Magnitude of Postprandial Spikes

As mentioned previously, glucose variability is something to avoid. Because rapid-acting insulin works slower than most forms of carbohydrate, postmeal glucose spikes often occur. When postmeal excursions (the rises that occur from premeal to the highest point after the meal) are excessive on a regular basis, both quality of daily life and long-term health can be compromised.

> No matter when the glucose peaks after a meal, it should show up on the CGM trend graph.

One of the really nice things about CGM is that it updates every 5 min. Unlike using fingersticks to capture postmeal glucose peaks, we don't have to guess when the glucose will hit its high point after a meal; it will appear on the CGM trend graph and downloaded reports no matter when it happens.

Case Study 3.3: Peter

The Dexcom Daily Trends graph (Fig. 3.6) is from a high school student named Peter who uses an insulin pump. Peter tends to bolus for his meals when he sits down to eat, and isn't sure what to do about the postmeal peaks because the glucose usually comes down to normal on its own a few hours later.

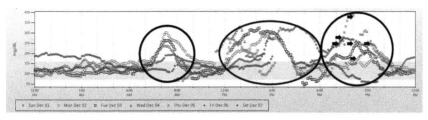

Figure 3.6—Peter's Daily Trends graph.

Observation: Peter is clearly "spiking" after most of his meals. After breakfast, his glucose rises to the 200–300 mg/dL [11–17 mmol/L] range before settling back to his target range before lunch. After lunch, he rises a similar amount and tends to stay at that level until after school. Because the time of his dinner varies, the postmeal pattern is less clear. By marking the high points each evening (see arrows), however, we can see that he rises to an average of ~250 mg/dL [14 mmol/L] after dinner before settling back to his target range by bedtime.

Conclusion: There is likely a timing mismatch between Peter's mealtime insulin and his carbohydrate digestion, and increasing his mealtime doses would only cause him to become hypoglycemic 2–4 h later (particularly after breakfast and dinner). With a goal of keeping his postmeal glucose <200 mg/dL [11 mmol/L] on a regular basis, he might benefit from taking his bolus insulin 15–20 min before eating. When this is not possible, he could make an effort to choose slower-digesting (low-glycemic-index) foods, or engage in some light physical activity right after eating.

Case Study 3.4: Lily

The Therapy Management Dashboard (from CareLink Pro) shown for Lily, a 26-year-old teacher, provides a definitive look at what takes place soon after she has her meals (Fig. 3.7). Remember, on this report, the moment the meal bolus is given is designated as time "0."

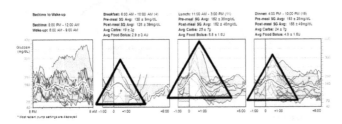

Figure 3.7—Lily's Therapy Management Dashboard.

Observation: Interestingly, Lily's glucose appears to start rising *before* she boluses for her meals. Her postbreakfast glucose peaks at ~160 mg/dL [9 mmol/L] on average. After lunch, she peaks at 220 mg/dL [12 mmol/L], and after dinner at 180 mg/dL [10 mmol/L].

Conclusion: Lily appears to be bolusing after she starts eating, and it is causing some significant postmeal glucose peaks, particularly after lunch. Lily would certainly benefit from giving her meal boluses before eating. She could also "split" her lunch (consume part at lunchtime, the remainder 1 or 2 h later, but give the full insulin dose before the first part) to provide a carb absorption pattern that matches her mealtime insulin absorption more closely.

Note that postmeal control problems are not limited to sharply rising glucose levels. Sometimes, glucose levels can drop soon after eating. So in a larger sense, trend graph tracings can be used to match the *timing* of mealtime insulin to different food types. This is sometimes referred to as "bolus sculpting."[43] It's like Goldilocks and the Three Boluses: the insulin can peak too early, too late, or just right. Consider the scenarios in Table 3.4.

Table 3.4—Postmeal Patterns and Insulin Timing

Insulin peak	On-screen pattern	Next time
Too early	Glucose drops 1–2 h postmeal, then rises afterward	Give insulin later, or extend the delivery of the bolus (if using a pump)
Too late	Glucose peaks very high 1–2 h postmeal, then drops toward target	Give insulin earlier
Just right	Slight rise 1–2 h postmeal, then settles into target range	Excellent! Lather, rinse, repeat

Case Study 3.5: Goldilocks

In the 6-h Dexcom trend graph shown in Fig. 3.8, Goldilocks gave her dinner bolus at 7 P.M. and ate a large Mexican-style meal that was high in fat and low-glycemic-index carbs 10 min later.

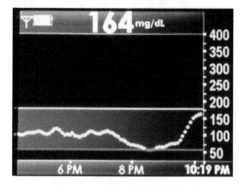

Figure 3.8—Goldilocks's trend graph.

Observation: Goldilocks saw her glucose drop low an hour after dinner. Confused, she ate some porridge and settled back to watch the Chicago Bears on *Monday Night Football*. To her surprise, her glucose rose quite high a few hours later.

Conclusion: The bolus Goldilocks took worked a little too soon for her slowly digesting meal. The next time she has Mexican-style food, she might benefit from giving her mealtime insulin after eating or, if she uses a pump, extending the delivery of the bolus.

Brilliant Insight 4.
Determining the Effectiveness of
Mealtime Insulin Doses

For those who take mealtime insulin, observing the glucose pattern 3–4 h after the meal provides a good assessment of the *magnitude* of the dose. Meal doses that are too low to cover the carbs in the meal will produce chronically elevated glucose levels 3–4 h later. Doses that are too high will have the opposite effect. Because unusual events can occur on any given day (e.g., miscounted carbs, changes in physical activity), it is best to look at several days of data at one time.

Case Study 3.6: Ira

The example in Fig. 3.9 is taken from Ira, an insulin pump user whose insulin-to-carbohydrate ratios (shown in the horizontal bars above the data above the graphs) are 1:9 at breakfast and lunch and 1:7 at dinner. In this Therapy Management Dashboard from CareLink Pro (a similar chart can be seen in the Sensor Overlay by Meal in CareLink Personal), the glucose can be observed following delivery of a meal bolus, designated as time "0."

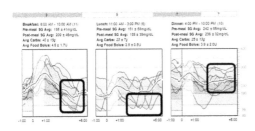

Figure 3.9—Ira's Therapy Management Dashboard.

Observation: Ira's glucose generally is within his target range 3–4 h after breakfast, below target following lunch, and above target following dinner.

Conclusion: Ira appears to need less insulin to cover his lunch and more to cover his dinner. He might consider discussing an adjustment to these doses (perhaps a 1:10 at lunch, and 1:6 at dinner) with his diabetes care team.

Case Study 3.7: Rhonda

In the Dexcom Patterns chart in Fig. 3.10, we can see the effects of meal-time insulin doses. Rhonda is on a multiple injection program and has her meals around 6–7 A.M., 11 A.M.–noon, and 5–6 P.M. daily, with a generous snack each night around 8 P.M. She takes fixed insulin doses of 5 units to cover breakfast and lunch, 8 units to cover dinner, and 4 units with her evening snack (adjusted based on her pre-meal/snack glucose level).

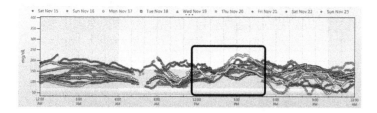

Figure 3.10—Rhonda's Patterns chart.

Observation: Rhonda's glucose levels following breakfast, dinner, and bedtime snack are typically within her target range 3–4 h after eating. Her postlunch glucose, however, rises and remains above target through most of the afternoon.

Conclusion: Rhonda's 5-unit lunch dose is no match for the carbs she is having at lunch. An increase in the insulin dose may be in order. A consultation with a dietitian regarding carb counting and portion estimation might also be beneficial.

Case Study 3.8: Oskar

Oskar is a very active 5-year-old boy who uses an insulin pump. He receives 1 unit of insulin for every 30 g carbohydrate at each meal and snack, with a correction factor of 140 mg/dL [7.8 mmol/L] and a target BG of 120 mg/dL [6.7 mmol/L]. A typical week of glucose values is shown in the Dexcom Daily Trends graph in Fig. 3.11.

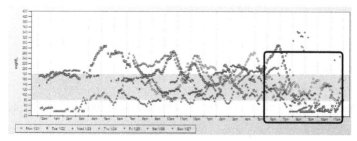

Figure 3.11—Oskar's Daily Trends graph.

Observation: Oskar's glucose levels are usually within his target range following his morning and afternoon meals and snacks, but he is often low following dinner. After the evening lows, he tends to have elevated glucose levels through the night.

Conclusion: Assuming that Oskar is not engaging in heavy exercise after dinner, it certainly looks as though he is receiving too much bolus insulin at dinnertime. The lows he has in the evening are probably contributing to the elevated readings later at night (following the daily tracings from 11 P.M. to 12 A.M. the next day verifies this to be the case). To prevent the lows after dinner, an adjustment to his dinnertime insulin-to-carbohydrate ratio is in order. Given that Oskar usually has 40 g carbohydrate at dinner and we need to raise his postdinner glucose by ~60–70 mg/dL [3.3–3.8 mmol/L], we can calculate the adjustment to his carb ratio this way: He currently receives 1.3 units to cover his 40 g dinner, but needs 0.5 units less (based on his correction factor). His new insulin-to-carbohydrate ratio can be calculated as follows: 40 g carbohydrate ÷ 0.8 units = a 1:50 insulin-to-carbohydrate ratio.

Brilliant Insight 5.
Quantifying the Correction Factor (Insulin Sensitivity)

In most cases, an individual's correction factor (or insulin sensitivity) is inversely related to the total amount of insulin taken per day.[44,45] Various formulaic approaches can be used to estimate the correction factor, but the formulas don't work for everyone. A number of factors can alter a person's daily insulin requirements and render an inappropriate correction factor when derived from a formula:

◆ A diet that is very high or very low in carbohydrates
◆ Production of even trace amounts of one's own insulin
◆ Unusual periods of stress or exercise
◆ Recent illness
◆ Use of medications that increase insulin sensitivity, such as thiazolidinediones
◆ Use of medications that reduce hepatic glucose output, such as biguanides
◆ Use of medications that reduce glucagon secretion, such as pramlintide, glucagon-like peptide-1 (GLP-1) analogs, and dipeptidyl peptidase-4 inhibitors

◆ Use of medications that increase glycosuria, such as sodium-glucose transporter-2 inhibitors

◆ Temporary use of steroid medications

In addition, many people find that their sensitivity to insulin varies by time of day. It is not uncommon to be more sensitive to correction doses delivered at night than to the same doses given during the day.

For these reasons, it is prudent to verify correction factors empirically based on sensor tracings. When a correction bolus is given without a concurrent meal dose, and no food is consumed (and no more bolus insulin given) for several hours, the resultant glucose level should indicate whether the correction factor is set properly. Of course, it is necessary to verify basal insulin doses before testing the correction formulas, because an incorrect basal setting will influence the outcome of a correction dose.

> Verify basal insulin doses before testing correction formulas.

Case Study 3.9: Jamie

Jamie was awakened in the middle of the night with a high glucose level. Based on his pump's bolus history, he delivered a correction bolus at 4:30 A.M. using his pump's bolus calculator. Another correction bolus was delivered mid-morning for an elevated reading. His pump is set for a target BG of 110 mg/dL [6.1 mmol/L] and a correction factor of 30 mg/dL [1.7 mmol/L] (1 unit is expected to lower his glucose 30 mg/dL [1.7 mmol/L]). His overnight and morning basal settings had been verified previously. His sensor tracing is shown in Fig. 3.12.

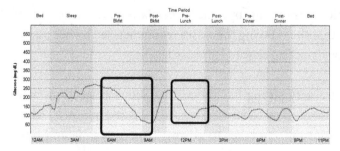

Figure 3.12—Jamie's sensor tracing.

Observation: Jamie's glucose dropped low ~4 h after he delivered his nighttime correction bolus. He ate to treat the low, and it appears that he rebounded up to a high level within 1 h. The correction bolus delivered midmorning brought the glucose down to target.

Conclusion: It is never a good idea to make setting changes based on a single event, but events like these are certainly grounds for discussion. Jamie has seen this sort of thing happen before—nighttime corrections that lead to lows. Jamie's nighttime correction factor may need to be increased to 35 or 40 mg/ dL [2–2.3 mmol/L]. His current correction factor (30 mg/dL [1.7 mmol/L]) appears to be working correctly during the day.

Case Study 3.10: Amy

Amy uses a Medtronic insulin pump and glucose sensor. Her correction factor is currently set at 45 mg/dL (2.5 mmol/L). She experiences hypoglycemia on almost a daily basis at various times of day.

Event Type Descriptions		
Event Types	%	Description
Rapid Falling Sensor Rate Of Change	68	Consider counseling your patient to take action to avoid hypoglycemia.
Bolus Wizard Food Bolus	55	Consider assessing the Bolus Wizard settings, counseling your patient on accurate carbohydrate counting, and/or the timing of insulin delivery with respect to carbohydrate intake.
Hyperglycemia Preceding Hypoglycemia	55	Consider assessing your patient's insulin sensitivity factors. Consider counseling your patient on the management of hyperglycemia.

Figure 3.13—Amy's Episode Summary report.

Observation: In the chart shown in Fig. 3.13, taken from a CareLink Pro Episode Summary report, more than half (55%) of Amy's hypoglycemic episodes for the previous month were preceded by hyperglycemia. A review of her Adherence report indicates that she is taking the doses recommended by her pump's bolus calculator when correcting elevated glucose levels.

Conclusion: There is a very strong likelihood that Amy's correction factor needs to be increased. Taking it up to 50 or 55 mg/dL [2.8 or 3 mmol/L] would reduce the amount of insulin she takes to correct hyperglycemia and likely would eliminate many of the subsequent lows.

Brilliant Insight 6.
Verifying the Effectiveness of Basal Insulin Doses

I have found CGM to be an *excellent* tool for fine-tuning basal insulin doses. Even when accuracy is in question, CGM's ability to detect rising and falling glucose levels is unparalleled. Because basal insulin's role is to achieve stability in glucose levels in the absence of digesting food, exercise, and active mealtime insulin, any significant rise or fall (>30 mg/dL [1.7 mmol/L] over a 4- to 6-h period) in a fasting/inactive state indicates a need to adjust the basal insulin dose.

Case Study 3.11: Natalie

The example in Fig. 3.14 is a Sensor Daily Overlay (from Medtronic Care-Link Personal) for Natalie, who is 5 months pregnant and uses an insulin pump. Because of her pregnancy, she is striving for very tight glucose control. Her last snack of the day is usually by 9 P.M., and a review of her logbook report indicated that she does not eat or bolus during the night.

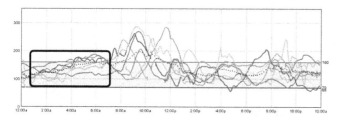

Figure 3.14—Natalie's Sensor Daily Overlay.

Observation: Natalie's glucose levels are rising an average of 60 mg/dL (3.3 mmol/L) during the night between 1 A.M. and 6. A.M.

Conclusion: It is very common for insulin needs to increase significantly during the second trimester of pregnancy. Natalie's basal insulin may need to be increased during the night. Given that it takes 1–2 h for a basal rate change to begin affecting glucose levels, an increase in her basal rate between 11 P.M. and 5 A.M. may be in order.

I've found that a *great* way for patients and health-care providers to communicate basal test results is via e-mailed photographs of CGM trend graph screens. It is important to capture the full test, so a 6- or 12-h display is usually necessary. It is also helpful (at least from my end) if the patient notes the time they last ate and took rapid-acting insulin before the test.

> A great way to communicate basal test results is to e-mail photographs of CGM trend graph screens.

Case Study 3.12: Jackie

In the Dexcom trend graph in Fig. 3.15, Jackie (who takes injections of glargine in the morning and rapid-acting insulin at meals) had a low-fat dinner at 7 P.M. and had no snacks (and took no more injections) after dinner.

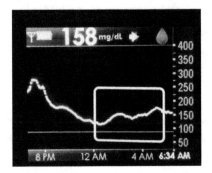

Figure 3.15—Jackie's trend graph.

Observation: Notice how Jackie's glucose was right on target around midnight (once her dinner insulin finished working), and then it rose steadily through most of the night.

Conclusion: Jackie's basal insulin, in this case her glargine, may need to be increased. It is also possible that her glargine is tapering off during the final 6–8 h of its action profile; she could talk with her health-care provider about splitting the dose: half in the morning, half in the evening.

Case Study 3.13: Stan

Stan, an insulin pump user, had a snack and took a bolus at 8 P.M., and then he fasted until morning (Fig. 3.16).

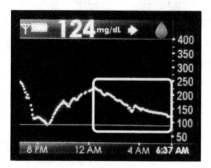

Figure 3.16—Stan's glucose levels.

Observation: Stan's glucose rose sharply following the snack. Then, after midnight, it dropped steadily until morning.

Conclusion: It appears that Stan has too much basal insulin working between midnight and ~7 A.M. To fix this, his basal rate would need to be reduced from 10 P.M. until 5 A.M. It is also possible that his snack bolus is too low. It would be worth observing the results of a few more evening snack scenarios to see whether this is a consistent issue.

Case Study 3.14: Karen

Karen, also an insulin pump user, decided to test her afternoon basal settings because of her frequent high readings before dinner. She ate breakfast (and bolused) at 8 A.M., and then she fasted and did not bolus or eat again until dinnertime (Fig. 3.17).

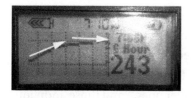

Figure 3.17—Karen's glucose reading.

Observation: The far-right side of the 6-h trend graph is around 7 P.M. Karen's glucose rose steadily from 1:30 P.M. until 5 P.M., and then it leveled off.

Conclusion: Karen appears to needs more basal insulin in the middle of the afternoon. Raising her basal rate between 12 noon and 3 or 4 P.M. should help to level out her glucose. Her basal appears to be set correctly in the late afternoon.

Let's take a look at one more overnight basal test (Fig. 3.18). The last bolus and meal was at 7 P.M. How would you interpret this? (The proposed solution follows.)

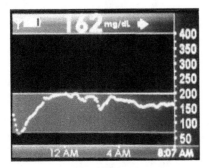

Figure 3.18—Karen's basal test.

Proposed Solution: The basal rate overnight looks fine. Even though it is slightly elevated through the night, it is steady, and that's what really matters when evaluating basal insulin. A very slight drop-off occurs between 1 A.M. and 6 A.M., but that is normal when the glucose is above renal threshold (180 mg/dL [10 mmol/L]).

Brilliant Insight 7.
Learning the Duration of the Insulin Action Curve

Knowing how long bolus insulin lasts is much more important than it sounds. Because all modern insulin pumps deduct bolus IOB or "active insulin" from correction or meal boluses whenever the pump's bolus calculator is used, knowing one's true duration of bolus action will ensure more accurate dosing and better control. Insulin action curves vary from person to person based on metabolic rate and subcutaneous absorption patterns. There is evidence that very large doses tend to have a longer action curve than smaller ones,[46] and those individuals with a rapid metabolism may have a shorter insulin action curve. Underestimation of the duration of insulin action can lead to chronic underestimation of IOB, and this sets pump users up for frequent overdosing and hypoglycemia. Overestimation can result in chronic underdosing of insulin and frequent hyperglycemia.

> Knowing the true duration of bolus action will ensure more accurate dosing and better control.

Although the insulin action curve may vary based on the volume of insulin taken, it can be helpful to determine each person's duration of bolus activity using a fairly typical dose. One way to do this is to examine the glucose response curve following administration of a correction dose only, as the glycemic effect of food may alter the postprandial glucose profile. To ensure that the glucose-lowering effect is from the bolus only, it is important to verify basal insulin doses before examining the duration of bolus action. Basal rates that are set too high can make boluses appear to last longer than they really do; basal rates that are too low can have the opposite effect.

Case Study 3.15: Jack

Below is a Medtronic CareLink sensor tracing for Jack, a 12-year-old boy whose parents administered a pump bolus for an elevated glucose level in the middle of the night (Fig. 3.19). A review of his logbook diary in CareLink Personal indicates that the bolus was taken at exactly 2:28 A.M., the same time a sensor calibration was performed. Incidentally, the same information can be found in the pump's bolus history. Jack's "active insulin time" is currently set for 3 h.

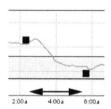

Figure 3.19—Jack's sensor tracing.

Observation: The SG begins dropping about 30 min after the bolus was given and "levels off" a little after 5:00 A.M.

Conclusion: Jack's bolus took ~3 h to finish working. The "active insulin time" setting in his pump looks as though it is set correctly.

Case Study 3.16: Kathryn

Kathryn takes multiple daily injections of insulin. Her glargine dose holds her steady overnight, but she is concerned about stacking her mealtime doses. She took an opportunity to wear a professional CGM to evaluate her insulin action profile. A segment of Kathryn's Dexcom Glucose Trend report is shown in Fig. 3.20. She took an injection of aspart insulin at 10:30 P.M. to cover a high reading and took no other injections (and did not eat) after that point.

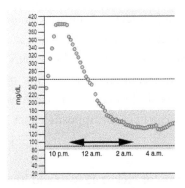

Figure 3.20—Kathryn's Glucose Trend report.

Observation: Kathryn's glucose began dropping shortly after the correction dose was administered and continued to fall until ~2:30 A.M.

Conclusion: In this instance, Kathryn's aspart insulin took about 4 h to finish working. She should take this into account when deciding whether or not to "correct" above-target glucose levels within 4 h of a previous injection.

Brilliant Insight 8.
Evaluating the Treatment of Hypoglycemia

Just about everyone with diabetes knows how good food tastes when you're low. Heck, even some nonfoods taste pretty good when we're low. Given that one's primal urge is to eat and continue eating until the symptoms go away, it is very common to see inappropriate and excessive treatment of hypoglycemia. For others, hypoglycemia is seen as a general nuisance, requiring unwanted calories. For these folks, undertreatment may be common. A quick look at individual-day trend graphs can provide insight into what happens *after* hypoglycemic events.

Case Study 3.17: Joanne

Joanne is an insulin pump user with a high degree of glucose variability. The hyperglycemic episodes chart in Fig. 3.21 (taken from a CareLink Pro Episode Summary report) for Joanne reveals the events that *preceded* her high readings.

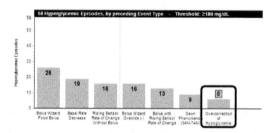

Figure 3.21 — Joanne's Episode Summary report.

Observation: Six times in the past month, Joanne had a high reading that came after a hypoglycemic event. Her hypoglycemic episodes chart showed that she had a total of six low glucose episodes in the past month.

Conclusion: Given that Joanne experienced high glucose following *every* episode of hypoglycemia, it is very likely that she is overtreating her lows. Perhaps she is consuming a slowly digesting form of carbohydrate and finds that she needs to treat several times until her symptoms dissipate. Or perhaps she is not taking insulin for the extra carbs she consumes (above and beyond the correct treatment). It is also possible that she is basing treatment on her CGM values, and because the CGM has an extended lag time in a state of hypoglycemia, she is treating multiple times unnecessarily. Regardless of the reason, education about (and adherence to) proper hypoglycemia treatment would likely solve this problem.

Case Study 3.18: Jerry

Jerry has type 2 diabetes and takes an injection of basal insulin only. Since the weather warmed up and he started to walk and work on his yard more, he has been experiencing frequent bouts of hypoglycemia. Fig. 3.22 is a 3-day Glucose Trend graph from a professional sensor session.

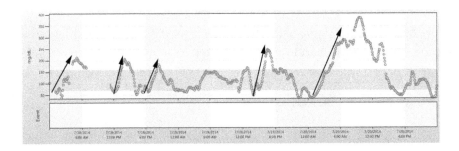

Figure 3.22—Jerry's Glucose Trend graph.

Observation: Jerry is experiencing hypoglycemia two or three times a day, at a variety of times. And every one of his *high* glucose events was preceded by hypoglycemia.

Conclusion: Jerry should talk with his health-care provider about possibly reducing his insulin dose during the warm-weather season. He also appears to be overtreating his lows, so a new and improved plan for treating hypoglycemia needs to be developed.

Brilliant Insight 9.
Titrating Incretin Mimetics

GLP-1 analogs and amylin can provide significant benefits to those who use them, particularly in the postprandial phase. By slowing gastric emptying and blocking pancreatic glucagon production, incretins have the potential to produce relatively flat, peakless glucose levels between meals, at least when a therapeutic dose is achieved. Titrating GLP-1 doses can be tricky. Take too little, and glucoses can continue to spike after meals. Take too much, and significant nausea can occur. By checking CGM trend graphs, it is possible to know when a therapeutically effective dose has been achieved without having to increase the dose unnecessarily.

Case Study 3.19: Angie

Angie started taking liraglutide, an injectable GLP-1, to help "smooth out" her type 2 diabetes. Her diabetes team set her up with a professional CGM to show her the effects of the medication. Her Dexcom trend graphs are shown in Figs. 3.23 and 3.24.

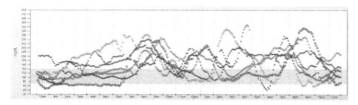

Figure 3.23—Angie's trend graph, 0.6 mg liraglutide.

Observation: It looks as though 0.6 mg of liraglutide has little (if any) effect on Angie's postmeal glucose levels. She continues to exhibit the peaks and valleys that are characteristic of accelerated gastric emptying.

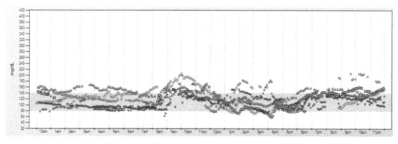

Figure 3.24—Angie's trend graph, 1.2 mg liraglutide.

Observation: Once her dose was increased to 1.2 mg, things really changed. Without altering her usual food and activity patterns, her glucose levels were considerably more stable, with minimal rise taking place after meals.

Conclusion: The CGM showed that 1.2 mg is a therapeutically effective dose for Angie. It saves her and her health-care team the trouble (time, cost, potential side effects) of increasing her dose further.

Brilliant Insight 10.
Discovering the Impact of
Lifestyle Events and Activities

CGM downloads allow users and their clinicians an opportunity to evaluate the effects of daily events so that effective management strategies can be developed. For example, what is the impact of the following:

◆ Various forms of exercise?
◆ Unusual stress?

◆ Illness or infection?

◆ Specific food types (such as restaurant meals)?

◆ Menstrual cycles?

◆ Work or school days versus off days?

It is necessary to have some information in addition to the CGM data to perform this type of evaluation. Records in the form of written logs; entries into smartphone apps; or event markers in meters, pumps, or CGM receivers can do the job just fine.

Because different forms of exercise can have varying effects on glucose levels, CGM provides an excellent tool for evaluating individual responses and formulating strategic adjustments. It can also motivate those who are starting an exercise program and who hope to see immediate therapeutic benefits.[47]

Case Study 3.20: Dana

Dana, who takes multiple daily injections of insulin, walks for exercise several times daily, including an early morning session most days of the week. She is careful to either take a snack or reduce her prior mealtime insulin dose by 25% if she plans to exercise. Still, she has blood glucose control problems surrounding her workouts. She agreed to keep track of her food, insulin, and exercise in her Dexcom receiver for 1 week so that she and her diabetes educator could look for a solution.

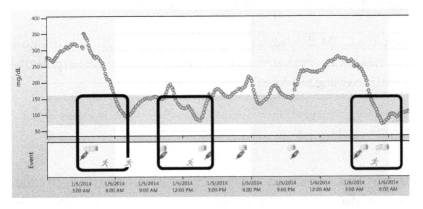

Figure 3.25—Dana's Glucose Trend graph.

Observation: In the Dexcom Glucose Trend graph (Fig. 3.25), we can see that Dana experiences a drop in her glucose following just about every bout of physical activity (denoted by the runners near the bottom of the chart). This is particularly true when she took a prior dose of insulin for a meal. The one time she exercised without a prior insulin dose (6 January 2014 at 7 A.M.), her glucose did not drop low afterward.

Conclusion: A 25% insulin dose reduction does not appear to be sufficient for preventing hypoglycemia when exercise takes place within the next couple of hours. Dana may need to experiment with a larger dose reduction, such as 33% or 50%.

Case Study 3.21: Ashley

Ashley, an insulin pump user, has carefully adjusted her basal insulin so that it holds her steady in a fasting state. However, she finds that she occasionally drops low overnight, even with a normal bedtime reading.

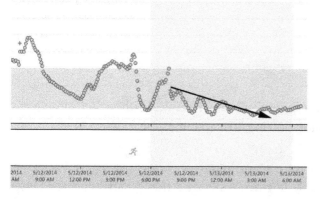

Figure 3.26—Ashley's Glucose Trend graph.

Observation: In the Dexcom Glucose Trend graph (Fig. 3.26), we can see that Ashley's glucose is close to normal 2–3 h after an evening workout, but it then starts to trail off.

Conclusion: Ashley may be experiencing *delayed onset hypoglycemia*—a drop in glucose that occurs several hours after intense exercise.[48,49] To prevent this drop, she could reduce the basal insulin delivered by her pump following intense workouts or consume a modestly sized, slowly digesting snack (without bolusing) before going to bed.

Case Study 3.22: Gary

Okay, I'll admit it. This is my own CGM report (Fig. 3.27). The data were collected in 2004, following an experimental trial using one of the first systems: MiniMed CGMS. The data were blinded to me, so I only had an opportunity to see the report after wearing the device for 3 days. This particular day stood out because I was late for an important afternoon meeting, had a flat tire on the way to the meeting, and discovered that my spare tire was also flat.

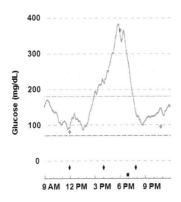

Figure 3.27—Gary's CGM report.

Observation: The stress response was unbelievable. Without consuming *any* food, my glucose rose almost 300 mg/dL [16 mmol/L].

Conclusion: Stress can have a powerful effect on glucose levels. Everyone, young and old, is susceptible to glucose swings if they let stress get the better of them. This experience motivated me to acquire some effective coping techniques for dealing with stressful situations.

Case Study 3.23: Andrea

A series of 1-month Glucose Trend graph reports were provided by an insulin pump user named Andrea to learn whether her menses were affecting her glucose levels (Fig. 3.28). Note that the x-axes indicate the date rather than time of day. The arrows near the bottom right of each chart indicate the onset of her menses for three consecutive months.

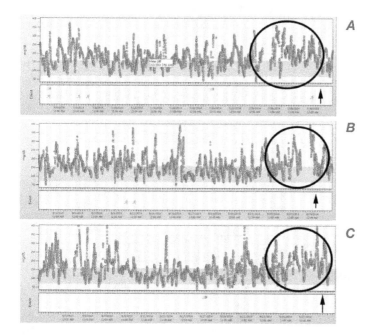

Figure 3.28—Andrea's Glucose Trend report, months 1 (*A*), 2 (*B*), and 3 (*C*).

Observation: Circles have been placed over the charts to point out that Andrea's glucose levels begin to rise 4–6 days before her menses, hit a high point 2–3 days prior, and return to normal at the start of her cycle.

Conclusion: Given that the elevated readings are occurring consistently several days before her menses, and the above-target values are not isolated to any specific time of day, Andrea and her diabetes care team could devise a plan to increase her basal insulin during these times. Because she uses an insulin pump, this result can be achieved through a series of temporary basal increases or by switching to a secondary basal pattern as her period approaches.

Case Study 3.24: Henry

Henry is retired and enjoys an active social life. On Friday and Saturday nights, he goes out with his buddies to shoot pool and indulge in bar food. He takes the same dose of glargine (basal) insulin at the same time every day for his type 2 diabetes. Still, his fasting readings vary considerably (Figs. 3.29 and 3.30).

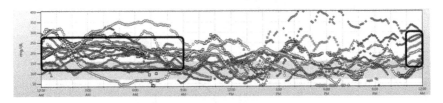

Figure 3.29—Henry's trend graph, Saturdays and Sundays.

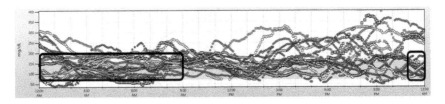

Figure 3.30—Henry's trend graph, weekdays.

Observation: In the Dexcom Daily Trends graphs, we can see how his overnight glucose levels compare on weekends versus weekdays. On weekends, his overnight glucose is generally in the 150–250 mg/dL [8–14 mmol/dL] range. On weekdays, he is nestled in the 80–160 mg/dL [4.5–9 mmol/L] range.

Conclusion: Given how Henry enjoys time out with his friends, it is probably not a good idea to discourage this tradition. If he wants to control his glucose better through the night, however, he might benefit from raising his glargine insulin dose on Friday and Saturday nights (being careful to watch for lows during the following day), or choose some lower-fat, lower-carb snacks at the bar.

Brilliant Insight 11.
Miscellaneous Shenanigans

People with diabetes are human, and humans sometimes do peculiar things. Occasionally, those peculiar things can undermine a health-care provider's best efforts to help patients improve their glycemic control. By combining CGM reports with data from pumps, apps, and written logs, the sources of undesirable glucose patterns can often be uncovered.

Case Study 3.25: John

John started using an insulin pump and CGM almost a year ago. Since then, his control has become progressively worse. His A1C is up a full point, and he still experiences regular bouts of hypoglycemia. Perhaps we can learn something from his CareLink Pro reports (Fig. 3.31).

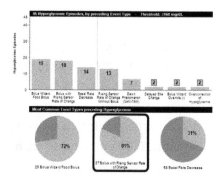

Figure 3.31—John's Episode Summary report.

Observation: John's Episode Summary report indicates that many hyperglycemic events coincide with a recent sensor "rise-rate" alert (Fig. 3.31). In fact, 81% of sensor rise-rate alerts are followed by a glucose level that is above target.

Conclusion: It appears that John may be ignoring his sensor alerts entirely. He probably would benefit from education on proper response to rise-rate alerts, such as engaging in physical activity or adjusting his bolus doses appropriately. Given the sheer number of rise-rate alerts (27 in the past week), he might also benefit from setting the threshold for the alert a bit higher so that he doesn't develop "sensor alert fatigue." For example, if his current rise-rate alert is set for 2 mg/dL/min [0.1 mmol/L/min], he could increase it to 3 mg/dL/min [0.17 mmol/L/min].

Case Study 3.26: Marley

Marley uses an insulin pump and was instructed during her training to change her infusion set every 2 days. Instead, she waits until her glucose becomes unstable. In this example (a 9-day Dexcom Glucose Trend report), we noted the dates of her infusion set changes (based on her pump's cannula prime history) with black triangles (Fig. 3.32).

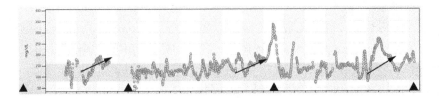

Figure 3.32—Marley's Glucose Trend report.

Observation: Notice how Marley's glucose takes an upswing on the third day of infusion set usage? Her glucose is mostly within range for the first 48 h, then starts to rise and becomes more erratic.

Conclusion: Marley would likely benefit from changing her infusion set every 48 h as she was originally instructed rather than waiting until problems set in. By being proactive rather than waiting for her glucose levels to rise, Marley should start to see more consistent glucose control.

Summary of Case Studies

Whew! That's a lot of brilliant insight (and a lot of graphs). Before you come down with a bad case of *datus overwhelmus*, don't forget that all of this information is *not* meant to be covered or accomplished in a single session. Whether you're caring for someone with diabetes or self-assessing your own data, try to glean a few insights at a time. For example, the first time you look at your (or your patient's) data, you might just want to focus on the basal insulin settings and perhaps look for patterns of hypoglycemia that require an immediate adjustment. It is usually best to take care of those two items before coming to conclusions about anything else. The next week (or month or scheduled appointment), you could focus on the effectiveness of mealtime doses and try to evaluate the duration of insulin action, and so on.

> Complete data analysis is rarely accomplished in a single session.

Consider the following sequence for CGM data analysis:

1. Look for patterns of hypoglycemia; examine pre- and post-hypoglycemia patterns

2. Evaluate basal insulin doses (particularly overnight) or effects of current medications
3. Evaluate bolus insulin doses (meal and correction) and insulin action curve
4. Measure postmeal peaks
5. Determine impact of lifestyle choices; examine data by day of week and time of month
6. Uncover potential educational needs

If exercise (or some other factor) plays a major role in one's life, that might take top priority. Rome wasn't built in a day, and fixing everything that might be wrong with a diabetes management program won't take place in a single session. Steady progress is what we're after. A few changes will move things in the right direction and give you an opportunity to evaluate and fine-tune further.

CHAPTER 4

Defeating the Downsides

G iven the plethora of ways one can benefit from both professional and personal CGMs, why would anyone *not* use them? Well, they do have a few drawbacks. This section addresses the challenges to using CGM and offers up strategies to help overcome (or at least minimize) these challenges. We'll end by presenting the "best of the best"—a series of take-home messages from leaders in the CGM field for ultimately getting the most out of the CGM experience.

OVERCOMING GENERAL CHALLENGES

In the one and only business course I took in college, the marketing professor emphasized that it's not enough to meet customer expectations. To truly succeed, you have to exceed expectations. "Nobody makes it big by overpromising and underdelivering," he said. To that end, it is important to set expectations at the proper level.

Although there are plenty of benefits to be had, CGM has its limits. A number of issues plague all CGM systems. Inserting the sensor can be a bit awkward and uncomfortable. Having something stuck on the skin all the time bothers some people. The tape may not stick well, and it can cause irritation for some people. There are periods of inaccuracy and occasional false alarms, and lag time always has to be considered. Transmitters and receivers require charging, and many people object to having to carry around an extra device. And finally, there are costs to consider. Even with good insurance coverage, copays and deductibles must be met. The strategies that follow can minimize the downsides, enhance CGM performance, and allow CGM to *exceed* expectations.

Strategy 1.
Calibrate Properly

Calibration plays an integral role in achieving the best possible system accuracy. All data generated by CGM are based on calibration values fed into the receiver. Feed the system well, and it will pay you back with better performance.

Health-care providers should place extra emphasis on teaching proper calibration procedures, particularly to users >55 years old.[5] Diabetes educators specializing in intensive management have reported that "lag time and calibrations were the most crucial teaching concepts for successful real-time CGM use."[50]

It is essential that accurate, timely calibration values are entered. For many users, this means breaking sloppy fingerstick monitoring habits that may have developed over the years. The "rules according to Hoyle" must be honored:

◆ Use a modern glucose meter with a good accuracy rating. Many older-generation meters are far less accurate than newer systems. Accuracy ratings usually can be found in the specifications section of the user manual. Look for a meter that is within 10% of lab values at least 95% of the time or that has a MARD of ≤6%.

◆ Use a blood sample from the fingertip (rather than an alternate site). Alternate-site readings, like CGM values, can lag a few minutes behind capillary blood measurements because they may contain interstitial fluid.

◆ Clean the finger and dry it completely before drawing the blood sample. Dirt, grease, and food residue can influence the glucose value significantly.

◆ Do not wipe the skin with alcohol before testing. Alcohol remaining on the skin can influence the blood sample.

◆ Apply a sufficient quantity of blood to the test strip. Some meters will generate false readings if too little blood is applied to the test strip.

◆ Make sure the meter is coded properly (if coding is required).

◆ Make sure the test strips are not expired and have been stored properly.

◆ If the fingerstick glucose value does not make sense (is much higher or lower than expected), check a second time just to confirm.

◆ If you doubt the reliability of the meter or strips, run a test using control solution. The result should fall within the range printed on the test strip package. Contact the meter manufacturer if you don't have control solution or if the one you have is past its expiration date.

Other suggestions when calibrating include the following:

◆ Calibrate when glucose levels are stable to avoid discrepancies related to lag time. Although this appears to be less of an issue with the Dexcom CGM,[51] as a general rule, if there are straight up or straight down arrows on your CGM display, postpone calibrating until the glucose is more stable.

◆ Calibrate at the times and frequency recommended by the device manufacturer. Generally, two to four calibrations daily works best. Calibrating too frequently or infrequently can hinder system performance.

◆ Enter the fingerstick BG value immediately after performing the test, lest you add to the lag-time discrepancy.

Even with optimal calibration, patience is a virtue. Many users find that sensor accuracy improves as the sensor ages. In particular, the first day of sensor usage tends to be the least accurate.[9] Once a few calibration points have been entered and a "wound" forms around the sensor, accuracy often improves significantly. However, sensors can fail to perform well even when calibrated properly, so fingersticks are still recommended for confirmation in most instances.

Strategy 2.
Minimize Nuisance Alerts

As discussed in Chapter 2, CGM systems offer many different types of alerts: high and low glucose, predictive high and low glucose, rapid rate of change, and general system alarms related to battery issues, sensor change reminders, calibration reminders, lost signals, and failed sensors. Although potentially useful from a diabetes management standpoint, the frequency of alerts can become disruptive and, if alerts are truly excessive or erroneous, may be ignored completely. For reference, see Aesop's "The Boy Who Cried Wolf."

The bottom line is that alerts will trigger appropriate action only if they are special, meaningful, and noticed. When alerts occur 20–30 times daily, they may no longer carry any significance for the user.

During the first few weeks of CGM usage, it is best to minimize the frequency of all alarms and alerts. Set the high alert at a level that is considered well above "desirable," and set the low alert at the lowest point of your acceptable glucose range. Set the alert "snooze" or "repeat" times for at least 2 h (high) and 1 h (low), and turn off the rate-of-change and predictive alerts entirely. Choose reminders and error message options that will produce the fewest possible disturbances.

Once you have a few weeks of CGM under your belt and are feeling comfortable with the nuances of the system, the high and low glucose levels can gradually be brought toward desired levels. As mentioned in Chapter 2, the fall rate and predictive low alerts may be beneficial to those making a concerted effort to ward off hypoglycemia, but set a relatively high fall-rate setting and a relatively short predictive-alert setting to minimize false alarms.

To avoid unnecessary reminder alerts, be proactive. Calibrate on a regular schedule, including before bedtime. This will prevent calibration reminders from disturbing you while you sleep. Also, charge devices that require charging on a regular basis. Doing so before the power drops to a very low level will prevent low-power alarms.

To ensure that the alerts draw the attention of the user (or user's caregiver), test the various alert volume levels as well as the vibrate option to see which works best. If possible, test them during sleep as well. Those who wear the receiver against their body, and hence under a blanket, usually do better using the vibrate feature than audible alerts.

If you're a very sound sleeper, consider the following creative options for enhancing the magnitude of alarms:

◆ Place the receiver on a nightstand in an empty drinking glass with the vibrate option enabled. For even more amplitude, put marbles in the glass.

◆ Place the receiver (in vibrate mode) on a smartphone that has an earthquake-detection (vibratory sensor) app installed.

◆ Put a baby monitor or walkie-talkie receiver near your bedside with the CGM receiver set to emit audible alerts. The second (linked) part of the baby monitor/walkie-talkie can be set at a very high volume.

Even with these types of magnifiers in place, you still may sleep through an alarm. If you are concerned about hypoglycemia during the night, setting an alarm clock to wake you for a quick glance at your receiver may still be your best option.

Strategy 3.
Manage the Sites

Discomfort, inflammation, and adhesion, oh my. Proper "site management" is important to both sensor performance and personal satisfaction with the system.

Let's discuss comfort first. Sensors are meant to reside in the subcutaneous fat—not the muscle, and certainly not within the skin (epidermal) layer itself. The fat layer has far fewer nerve endings than the tissues above and below, so choose a "fleshy" area for inserting sensors. In very lean individuals, including young children and athletes, the upper buttock can serve as an excellent sensor site. Note that the upper buttock was not evaluated as a sensor site before FDA approval of the CGM devices, but overall user experience using this area has been quite positive.

Users who have tried placing sensors on their upper buttocks have reported good sensor performance.

Avoid scar tissue, locations where tight clothing may be worn (such as waistbands), and places that might be rubbed or struck often. Although the sensors are composed of a flexible material, pressure on (or contact with) the sensor housing can cause discomfort. Follow the instructions that come with the sensor insertion device, and insert the introducer needle rapidly and at the recommended angle. When proper insertion procedures are followed, the degree of discomfort should be minimized. Those who are overly anxious about the sensor insertion procedure or have a particularly low pain threshold may discuss skin-numbing options with their health-care team.

Unlike insulin pump infusion sets, which release insulin into the body, sensors are relatively benign. It is our clinical experience that infections and inflammation at sensor sites are extremely rare. It is still best, however, to clean and dry the site and rotate sensor sites to allow proper healing of the skin surface and subcutaneous tissues. Alternating body parts is fine but not required; moving the sensor 1–2 inches (3–5 centimeters) will do the job (see the rotation chart in Table 4.1).

Table 4.1—Rotation Chart

Left side	Right side
1 2 3	9 8 7
4 5 6	12 11 10

In the event that your sensor site exhibits any of the following, remove the sensor and contact your health-care provider:

◆ Pain, tenderness, or soreness
◆ Redness around the site
◆ Itching or irritation
◆ Inflammation
◆ A hard bump
◆ Release of pus
◆ A foul odor

Additionally, CGM users may develop an allergy or sensitivity that may cause a rash or other changes to the appearance or texture of the skin. To minimize contact between the sensor adhesive patch and the skin surface, a number of options are available. Placing one or two adhesive dressings (such as IV3000 or Tegaderm) on the skin before inserting the sensor, and inserting the sensor directly through the dressings, often will alleviate the problem. For particularly stubborn allergies, a thicker hydrocolloidal dressing, such as Band-Aid Tough Pads (Johnson & Johnson) made with Compeed Moisture Seal technology, can do the trick. In extreme cases, to prevent local reactions, it may be necessary to apply a steroidal spray or ointment to the skin prior to inserting the sensor. Because the performance of the sensor may be affected by inserting through an adhesive, each user must weigh the pros and cons of using a skin barrier. CGM users should work with their health-care team, including a dermatologist, to find an optimal solution.

For those who use an insulin pump, juggling pump infusion sites and sensor sites can be a challenge. Recent research, however, has suggested that it may not be necessary to keep pump and sensor sites separated by any particular distance.[52] Because the change frequency is different for pump and sensor sites, it is best to ensure that the tape for each does not overlap with the other.

Speaking of tape, let's address the issue of adhesion. Adhesion is important not only for comfort but also for sensor performance. Movement of the sensor below the skin may cause irritation, poor signal transmission, and erroneous glucose values. Having a sensor peel off the skin because of adhesion failure wastes time and money. Although most manufacturers will replace sensors that peel off prematurely, it can be frustrating to have to insert a new sensor and repeat the warm-up process.

Adhesives vary from sensor to sensor, but all work best when the sensor site is clean and free of oils, creams, and ointments. It is also best to place the sensor on a site that does not twist or stretch a great deal, as this puts strain on the adhesive.

Dexcom sensor adhesive generally holds the sensor in place for about a week. Those who choose to disregard the manufacturer's recommendation and use their sensors beyond 7 days will almost always need to apply extra tape over the adhesive part of the sensor. We have found it best to not cover the transmitter, as this can cause moisture to accumulate under the tape. Ideally, start with a 3 inch × 4 inch (or larger) adhesive dressing, cut a rectangle in the center to match the size of the transmitter housing, and place it in one piece over the sensor adhesive. Tegaderm (3M), IV3000 (Smith & Nephew), and OPSITE FLEXFIX (Smith & Nephew; Fig. 4.1) are good options. IV3000, in particular, seems to minimize irritation thanks to its "breathable" design.

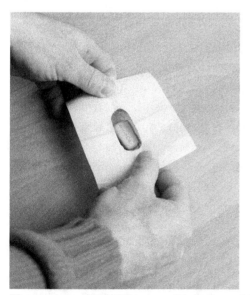

Figure 4.1—OPSITE tape with hole cut to secure sensor adhesive.

Medtronic Enlite sensors come with their own adhesive overbandages with a precut hole in the center, but these patches are small and do not cover the entire transmitter. It is easy to snag the transmitter and pull the entire sensor out when the transmitter is not sealed against the skin. To prevent movement of the sensor and accidental pullout, we have found it helpful to apply extra tape over the entire sensor-transmitter apparatus soon after inserting.

One other potential site issue involves the metal component of the sensors themselves. Although the amount of metal is not enough to trigger airport metal detectors and X-ray equipment, there may be enough to cause damage if the sensor is worn in or around magnetic resonance imaging (MRI) equipment. All device manufacturers recommend removing the sensor before undergoing an MRI. See the Appendix for a detailed list of products for sensor site management.

Strategy 4.
Ensure Proper Transmission and Reception

Skipped data and lost signals can get in the way of daily sensor use and be another source of frustration for the user. To minimize the incidence of skipped data, particularly with Medtronic systems, the user should wear the receiver (pump or Guardian) on the same side of their body as the sensor. This reduces water interference caused by the body itself (radio signals from the transmitters do not travel well through water). Make sure the transmitter is properly charged and seated or attached to the sensor, and report any transmission or reception problems to the manufacturer. Transmission issues may be a sign that the transmitter is worn out or defective and requires replacement.

CGM transmitter use during air travel is open to debate. The device manufacturers warn against using CGM on aircraft, and most airlines ask that transmitters be placed in suspend mode during air travel. However, the range (and frequency) of CGM transmitters should have no bearing on airline equipment. To my knowledge, there is no evidence to suggest that use of CGM transmitters during air travel causes any interference with aircraft equipment or issues with sensor performance.

Strategy 5.
Reduce Out-of-Pocket Costs

The upfront cost for a CGM system and the ongoing expenses for disposable sensors and transmitters are beyond the reach of many people. However, health insurance coverage for CGM is improving all the time. As of the publication of this book, more than 90% of private health plans and some public plans offer some degree of coverage. CGM is usually considered durable medical equipment

(DME) and is subject to the same deductibles and copays as other types of DME (including pumps and infusion sets or meters and test strips). Every CGM company has a team of specialists dedicated to helping customers obtain maximum coverage. *Let the manufacturer work on your behalf.* They know exactly the right things to ask, say, and provide to verify and secure coverage for CGM.

Factors that may help to support coverage of CGM in people with type 1 or type 2 diabetes include the following:

- A history of hypoglycemia, documented in the physician's chart or records or in a meter download
- Presence of hypoglycemia unawareness
- Highly variable BG levels
- Suboptimal HbA$_{1c}$
- Frequent BG monitoring
- Completion of diabetes self-management education

If you are denied coverage for CGM, following through with an appeal gives another opportunity to explain your case and may result in a reversal of the insurance company's original decision. If difficulties with your health plan persist, and switching or upgrading plans is not an option, several online resources may help:

- JDRF has a blog site that offers useful tips regarDing insurance coverage for CGM at http://jdrf.org/blog/2008/insurance-coverage-for-continuous-glucose-monitors
- Excellent sample letters for establishing medical need can be found at www.diabeteshealth.com/read/2009/02/27/6096/sample-request-for-cgm-insurance-coverage
- For Additional Resources for CGM Insurance Coverage, including a detailed list of plans that cover CGM, visit the CGM Anti-Denial Campaign website at http://cgm-antidenial.ning.com
- Dexcom has an online list, by region, of insurance plans that cover CGM for people with type 1 and type 2 diabetes at www.dexcom.com/reimbursement
- Medtronic provides a reimbursement guide for health care professionals regarding patient CGM training and data analysis services at www.professional.medtronicdiabetes.com/reimbursement-lookup-tool

OVERCOMING DEVICE-SPECIFIC CHALLENGES

Each CGM device has its own unique set of quirks and idiosyncrasies. The following are strategies developed by our team of CGM-wearing and -training certified diabetes educators, with input from manufacturers' clinical experts and a host of colleagues in the diabetes community:

Medtronic Enlite Insider Tips

Try the following before inserting the sensor:

◆ Refrigerate the sensors during storage. This helps to ensure that they stay fresh and may extend their life past the expiration date printed on the packaging.

◆ Use an alcohol swab to exfoliate the skin where the sensor adhesive will be placed. This removes dead surface skin cells and promotes better adhesion.

◆ Use the latest-model transmitter whenever possible. Older, out-of-warranty transmitters may have metallic connector contacts that are slightly bent or misaligned. This can cause a sawtooth appearance in the trend graph tracings.

◆ Make sure transmitters are *fully* charged before using them. The very first time the transmitter is charged, full charging may take up to 12 h. After the first use, a full recharge takes about 20–30 min. Wait until a constant green light appears on the charger. When not using the transmitter, leave it in the charger so that the power does not drain completely.

Try the following during sensor insertion (see Fig. 4.2):

◆ To minimize "rocker" motions of the sensor or transmitter, position the inserter so that the transmitter will be above (north of) the sensor once it is connected.

◆ Before loading the sensor into the inserter, handle it only by the base. Otherwise, the introducer needle can bend accidentally.

◆ When loading the sensor into the inserter, make sure the flap of tape that will go over the transmitter is folded down and not sticking out.

If the flap is sticking out, it could adhere to the inserter and pull the whole sensor out when the inserter is removed.

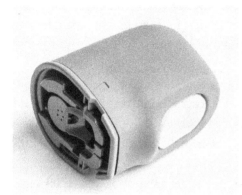

Figure 4.2—Medtronic Enlite Serter.

◆ When inserting the sensor, press and release the protruding part of the green button quickly. Then, hold the inserter in place for 15–20 sec. Press and hold the green button while removing the inserter.

◆ Use a light touch when inserting the sensor. The insertion device just needs to rest on the surface of the skin; there is no need to press into the skin.

◆ When pulling the needle housing off the sensor, hold the base of the sensor at the top and bottom, not on the sides. Holding the sides will lock the needle housing in place (see Fig. 4.3).

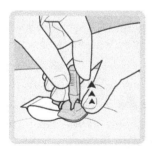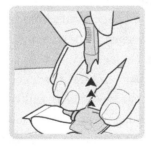

Figure 4.3—Proper handling of the needle housing. Image used with permission of Medtronic Diabetes.

◆ If there is often a weak signal or very poor accuracy at the beginning of sensor usage, consider leaving the sensor in overnight before connecting the transmitter and "starting" the sensor.

◆ After connecting the transmitter, gently fold the flap of tape over the body of the transmitter. Don't pull the flap too tightly.

Try the following after the sensor is in place:

◆ When calibrating, make sure the Cal Factor is between 3 and 8 to avoid generating a Cal Error message (Cal Factor = BG ÷ ISIG, found in the sensor status screen). Repeated "cal errors" may generate a sensor failure alert.

◆ If you need to calibrate a second time to get a sensor back on track (due to a Cal Error message), wait at least 15 min.

◆ When a Thresh Suspend alert occurs, check your glucose with a fingerstick meter and treat with rapid-acting carbohydrate if necessary. Food will help raise the glucose much faster than suspending basal insulin. When your glucose has risen to a safe level, cancel the alert and resume basal insulin delivery. Do not leave the pump in "suspend" mode, as this may cause an undesired glucose rise a few hours later.

Dexcom G4 Insider Tips

Consider the following tips when using Dexcom:

◆ Make absolutely sure that the transmitter is secured below both side arms on the sensor housing (i.e., listen for a double click when attaching the transmitter). If only one arm is holding the transmitter down, the contact between the sensor and transmitter may be tenuous, and water can enter the space.

◆ Acetaminophen (a pain and fever reducer found in Tylenol products and many cold and flu medicines) will cause the Dexcom sensor to generate abnormally high readings for several hours. If you must use acetaminophen, revert to routine fingersticks until the sensor returns to normal performance—typically 4–8 h later.

◆ Dexcom receivers are very water sensitive, even when the charging port is covered by the slide piece. It only takes a drop of water entering the "guts" of the receiver to damage it permanently. Avoid exposing the receiver to splashing, spraying, and undue moisture.

◆ Be careful when inserting the download/charging cable into the side port on the receiver. Pushing too hard or twisting the connector can cause the housing to come loose. Align the cable connector properly (it will be top-side down) and insert *gently*.

INGREDIENTS FOR SUCCESS

Throughout this book, we've discussed many strategies for optimizing CGM use. We've presented ways to improve real-time decision making and shared techniques for improving overall diabetes management through retrospective analysis of CGM data. In this chapter, we focused on overcoming the various shortcomings of CGM systems—hurdles we all hope will be minimized as CGM technology continues to improve.

Now it's time to take a step back and see the bigger picture. Let's put it all together in a series of concise best practices for ensuring CGM success.[53,54]

1. Enter CGM use with the right expectations. Whether you're using CGM on an ongoing (personal) or temporary (professional/loaner) basis, understand the limitations of the current systems. Experts have found that CGM users are more successful when they learn about and understand the technology *before* initiating use.[55] Use CGM to your advantage, but don't expect it to solve everything.

2. If you're going to use CGM personally, use it regularly. Research spearheaded by JDRF has shown that those who use CGM on a daily basis (at least 6 days/week) are much more likely to experience the key benefits: fewer and less severe hypoglycemic events, improvements in A1C, and less variability in glucose levels. Those who don't use CGM on a consistent basis may benefit intermittently but are less likely to see long-term improvements in glucose control or significant reductions in hypoglycemia.[51,56]

3. Calibrate appropriately. As discussed extensively in this chapter, CGM's performance hinges on timely and accurate calibrations. Feed it well, and it will function at its best.

4. Capitalize on the alerts. One of the key benefits of CGM is the alert system that allows users to reverse highs and lows before they become too severe.

Set the alerts so that they are meaningful, not a menace. This is particularly important during the first several weeks of CGM usage. (For more details, see Chapter 2, pages 25–33.)

5. Look at the receiver regularly, but don't become obsessed. Research has shown that those who benefit the most from CGM usage look at their data on a frequent basis.[57] But there is such a thing as too much information. Checking excessively can be counterproductive and can lead to too many knee-jerk reactions. I have found that checking the receiver about once an hour seems to achieve a nice balance.

6. Analyze the data, but do so with a narrow focus. Technology is only valuable if it is utilized effectively. Whether you're a CGM user or a health-care professional, evaluating the data and making strategic adjustments are very important. Given the complexity and sheer volume of data generated by CGM software, it is necessary to have a game plan—an *agenda*—when reviewing and analyzing the reports. (For more details, see Chapter 3, pages 46–47.)

7. Adjust therapy based on trends and patterns. You know the saying, "On any given day, anything can happen." Even my hometown Philadelphia 76ers can win a basketball game once in a while. When they do, it would be foolhardy to assume that they're the best team in the NBA. Likewise, most changes to a diabetes management program should not be based on single events, but on regular and repeated patterns—the kind that show up on the multiple-day trend graph and statistical reports.

8. Do not overreact to the real-time data. This is a follow-up to the idea of not looking at the receiver too often. Consider the full picture when adjusting to momentary high and low readings. For those who take insulin at mealtimes, IOB (bolus insulin on board) should always be taken into account. When glucose levels are falling, consider food that might still be digesting. And the prolonged effects of exercise, illness, medications, and other factors need to be incorporated into one's decision making. Diabetes management is never simple. (For more details, see Chapter 2.)

THE OUTLOOK IS BRIGHT

The trend in CGM product development is very positive. New-generation systems appear every couple of years, sporting better sensor accuracy, stronger transmitters, and improved system functionality. There is a growing movement toward linking the sensors with insulin pumps and smartphones, thus eliminating the need to carry a receiver. There is also a trend toward smaller equipment with features that mimic consumer electronics. And as research continues to demonstrate the safety and efficacy of CGM, public and private third-party payers are covering the costs of CGM on a more comprehensive and consistent basis.

Much more important than cutting costs and superficial product features is the integration of CGM with hormone-delivery devices (pumps) that mimic the function of a healthy pancreas in the management of diabetes. By taking data from the glucose sensor and translating it into the infusion of hormones that lower glucose (insulin), raise glucose (glucagon), and modulate the appearance of glucose in the bloodstream (amylin), a closed-loop "artificial pancreas" is well within reach.

Until then, take advantage of the technology that is available *now*. CGM systems are far from perfect. But what they do offer us, as people living with diabetes and the health-care professionals who treat them, is an opportunity to take diabetes management to a whole new level.

Helpful Products for Sensor Site Management

Antiseptics (for those with a history of cellulitis, staph, or compromised immunity)
- Hibiclens
- Betadine
- Povidone-iodine wipes
- BZK towelettes (benzalkonium chloride)

Topical Numbing (generally not necessary; only to be used as needed)
- Ice in a paper cup
- Numby Stuff
- LMX4 Cream
- EMLA Cream

Barrier Wipes
- IV Prep
- Skin-Prep
- Bioclusive
- Bard Protective Barrier Film

Adhesive Aids
Preinsertion solutions
- Skin-Tac-H
- Skin Bond
- Tincture of benzoin
- Hypercare 20% AlCl antiperspirant
- Mastisol

Postinsertion overtapes/dressings
- OpSite IV 3000
- Tegaderm
- DuoDERM
- PolySkin
- Hypafix
- Transpore
- Micropore
- Mefix

Anti-Itch/Allergy (applied to skin prior to insertion)
- Tough Pads
- Benadryl itch relief spray
- Hydrocortisone lotion
- Caladryl lotion

Solvents (for removing adhesive more easily)
- Baby oil
- Uni-Solve
- Detachol
- Remove Adhesive Remover

Topical Antibacterials
(if redness, inflammation, or discharge is noted upon removal of the sensor)
- Bacitracin
- Neosporin
- Polysporin
- Bactroban cream

*Thank you to the Phoenix Children's Hospital for contributing exensively to this list.

This list provides product information but does not imply an endorsement by the American Diabetes Association.

References

1. Battelino T, et al. Effect of continuous glucose monitoring on hypoglycemia in type 1 diabetes. *Diabetes Care* 2011;34:795–800

2. Raccah D, et al. Incremental value of continuous glucose monitoring when starting pump therapy in patients with poorly controlled type 1 diabetes: the RealTrend study. *Diabetes Care* 2009;32(12):2245–2250

3. Chitaya L, Zisser H, Jovanovic L. Continuous glucose monitoring during pregnancy. *Diabetes Technol Ther* 2009;11(Suppl. 1):S105–S111

4. Yoo HJ, et al. Use of a real-time continuous glucose monitoring system as a motivational device for poorly controlled type-2 diabetes. *Diab Res Clin Pract* 2008;82:73–79

5. Allen N, Fain J, Braun B, Chipkin SR. Continuous glucose monitoring in non–insulin-using individuals with type 2 diabetes: acceptability, feasibility, and teaching opportunities. *Diabetes Technol Ther* 2009;11(3):151–158

6. Kropff J, et al. Accuracy of two continuous glucose monitoring systems: a head-to-head comparison under clinical research centre and daily life conditions. *Diabet Obes Metab* 2014. doi:10.1111/dom.12378. Epub 10 Sept 14

7. Freckmann G, Pleus S, Link M, Zschornack E, et al. Technology Society performance evaluation of three continuous glucose monitoring systems: comparison of six sensors per subject in parallel. *J Diabet Sci Technol* 2013;7(4):842–853

8. Luijf YM, et al. Accuracy and reliability of continuous glucose monitoring systems: a head-to-head comparison. *Diabetes Technol Ther* 2013(15):721–726

9. Matuleviciene V, et al. A clinical trial of the accuracy and treatment experience of the Dexcom G4 sensor (Dexcom G4 System) and Enlite sensor (Guardian REAL-Time System) tested simultaneously in ambulatory patients with type 1 diabetes. *Diabetes Technol Ther* 2014;16(11):1–9

10. Calhoun P, Lum J, Beck RW, Kollman C. Performance comparison of the Medtronic Sof-Sensor and Enlite glucose sensors in inpatient studies of individuals with type 1 diabetes. *Diabetes Technol Ther* 2013;15(9): 758–761

11. Damiano E, et al. A comparative effectiveness analysis of three continuous glucose monitors: the Navigator, G4Platinum, and Enlite. *J Diabetes Sci Technol* 2014;8(4):699–708

12. Enlite Sensor Performance for the MiniMed 530G Insulin Pump [clinical appendix]. Minneapolis, MN, Medtronic Inc., 2014

13. Pleus S, et al. Performance evaluation of a continuous glucose monitoring system under conditions similar to daily life. *J Diabet Sci Technol* 2013;7(4):833–841

14. Bailey T, Chang A, Christiansen M. Clinical accuracy of a continuous glucose monitoring system with an advanced algorithm. *J Diabetes Sci Technol* 2014. Available from http://dst.sagepub.com/content/early/2014/11/03/1932296814559746. Epub 3 Nov 14

15. Dexcom G4 Platinum [user's guide]. San Diego, CA, Dexcom Inc., 2012

16. Kamath A, Aarthi M, Brauker J. Analysis of time lags and other sources of error of the DexCom SEVEN Continuous Glucose Monitor. *Diabetes Technol Ther* 2009;11(11):689–695

17. Boyne MS, Silver DM, Kaplan J, Saudek CD. Timing of changes in interstitial and venous blood glucose measured with a continuous subcutaneous glucose sensor. *Diabetes* 2003;52:2790–2794

18. Keenan DB, et al. Accuracy of the Enlite 6-day glucose sensor with Guardian and Veo calibration algorithms. *Diabetes Technol Ther* 2012;14(3):225–231

19. Hammon PJ, et al.; on behalf of the Association of British Clinical Diabetologists (ABCD) and endorsed by the British Society for Paediatric Endocrinology and Diabetes (BSPED). ABCD position statement on continuous glucose monitoring: use of glucose sensing in outpatient clinical diabetes care. *Pract Diab Int* 2010;27(2):66–68

20. Liebl A, Henrichs H.; for the Continuous Glucose Monitoring Working Group of the Working Group Diabetes Technology of the German Diabetes Association. Continuous glucose monitoring: evidence and consensus statement for clinical use. *J Diabetes Sci Technol* 2013;7(2):500–519

21. Blevins TC, et al. Statement by the American Association of Clinical Endocrinologists Consensus Panel on Continuous Glucose Monitoring. *Endocr Pract* 2010;16(5)

22. American Diabetes Association. Standards of medical care in diabetes—2014. *Diabetes Care* 2014;37(Suppl. 1):S1–S93

23. Geddes J, Schopman J, Zammitt NN, Frier BM. Prevalence of impaired awareness of hypoglycaemia in adults with type 1 diabetes. *Diabet Med* 2008;25(4):501–504

24. Weber K, Lohmann T, Busch K, Donati-Hirsch I, Riel R. High frequency of unrecognized hypoglycaemias in patients with type 2 diabetes is discovered by continuous glucose monitoring. *Exp Clin Endocrinol Diabetes* 2007;115:491–494

25. Smith C, et al. Hypoglycemia unawareness is associated with reduced adherence to therapeutic decisions in patients with type 1 diabetes. *Diabetes Care* 2009;32(7):1196–1198

26. Wolpert HA. Use of continuous glucose monitoring in the detection and prevention of hypoglycemia. *J Diabet Sci Technol* 2007;1:146–150

27. Buckingham B, Wilson D, Lecher T, Hanas R, et al. Duration of nocturnal hypoglycemia before seizures. *Diabetes Care* 2008;31(11):2110–2112

28. Bode B, et al. Alarms based on real-time sensor glucose values alert patients to hypo- and hyperglycemia: the Guardian continuous monitoring system. *Diabetes Technol Ther* 2004;6:105–113

29. Battelino T, et al. Effect of continuous glucose monitoring on hypoglycemia in type 1 diabetes. *Diabetes Care* 2011;34:795–800

30. Leelarathna L, et al. Restoration of self-awareness of hypoglycemia in adults with long-standing type 1 diabetes: hyperinsulinemic-hypoglycemic clamp substudy results from the HypoCOMPaSS trial. *Diabetes Care* 2013;36(12):4063–4070

31. Colberg, S. *Exercise and Diabetes: A Clinician's Guide to Prescribing Physical Activity.* Alexandria, VA, American Diabetes Association, 2013

32. Choudhary P, et al. Insulin pump therapy with automated insulin suspension in response to hypoglycemia. *Diabetes Care* 2011;34:2023–2025

33. Bergenstal R, et al. Threshold-based insulin-pump interruption for reduction of hypoglycemia. *N Engl J Med* 2013;369:224–232

34. Pearson I, Bergenstal R. Fine-tuning control: pattern management versus supplementation. *Diabetes Spectr* 2001;14(2):76

35. Ritholz M, et al. Psychosocial factors associated with use of continuous glucose monitoring. *Diabetic Med* 2010;27(9):1060–1065

36. Clark D, King AB. Basal glucose testing: a carbohydrate free meal does not equal meal omission. *Diabetes* 2010;59(Suppl. 1):A554

37. Nathan D, Kuenen J, Borg R, Zheng H, et al. Translating the A1C assay into estimated average glucose values. *Diabetes Care* 2008;31:1473–1478

38. Martin DD, Davis EA, Jones TW. Acute effects of hyperglycaemia in children with type 1 diabetes mellitus: the patient's perspective. *J Pediatr Endocrinol Metab* 2006;19(7):927–936

39. Liu Y, Li Y-Y, Cai H, Zhang X. The relationship between glycemic variability and macrovascular and microvascular complications in type 2 diabetes. Abstract presented at the American Diabetes Association 71st Scientific Sessions, San Diego, CA, 24–28 June 2011; abstract 2205-PO

40. Su G, et al. Impact of admission glycemic variability, glucose, and glycosylated hemoglobin on major adverse cardiac events after acute myocardial infarction. *Diabetes Care* 2013;36(4):1026–1032

41. Hirsch I, Brownlee M. Beyond hemoglobin A1C—need for additional markers of risk for diabetic microvascular complications. *JAMA* 2010;303(22):2291–2292

42. American Diabetes Association. Standards of medical care in diabetes—2015. *Diabetes Care* 2015;38(Suppl. 1)S1–S93

43. King A. Continuous glucose monitoring-guided insulin dosing in pump-treated patients with type 1 diabetes: a clinical guide. *J Diabet Sci Technol* 2012;6(1):191–203

44. Hagnas R. *Type 1 Diabetes—a Guide for Children, Adolescents, Young Adults and Their Caregivers.* New York, NY, Marlowe & Company, 2005

45. King A, Armstrong D. A prospective evaluation of insulin dosing recommendations in patients with type 1 diabetes at near normal glucose control: bolus dosing. *J Diabetes Sci Technol* 2007;1(1):42–46

46. Gagnon-Auger M, et al. Dose-dependent delay of the hypoglycemic effect of short-acting insulin analogs in obese subjects with type 2 diabetes—a pharmacokinetic and pharmacodynamic study. *Diabetes Care* 2010;33(12):2502–2507

47. Riddell M, Perkins B. Exercise and glucose metabolism in persons with diabetes mellitus: perspectives on the role for continuous glucose monitoring. *J Diabet Sci Technol* 2009;3(4):914–923

48. Diabetes Research in Children Network (DirecNet) Study Group. Impaired overnight counterregulatory hormone responses to spontaneous hypoglycemia in children with type 1 diabetes. *Pediatr Diabetes* 2007;8(4):199–205

49. Maran A, et al. Continuous glucose monitoring reveals delayed nocturnal hypoglycemia after intermittent high-intensity exercise in nontrained patients with type 1 diabetes. *Diabetes Technol Ther* 2010;12(10): 763–768

50. Messer L, et al. Educating families on real time continuous glucose monitoring. *Diabetes Educator* 2009;35(1):124–135

51. Mahalingam A, Garcia A, Kamath A. Calibration of a continuous glucose monitor (CGM): effect of glucose rate of change. Paper presented at the 71st Scientific Session of the American Diabetes Association, San Diego, CA, 24–28 June 2011(0888-P)

52. O'Neal D, Adhya S, Jenkins A, Ward G, et al. Feasibility of adjacent insulin infusion and continuous glucose monitoring via the Medtronic Combo set. *J Diabet Sci Technol* 2013;7(2):381–388

53. Juvenile Diabetes Research Foundation Continuous Glucose Monitoring Study Group. Factors predictive of use and of benefit from continuous glucose monitoring in type-1 diabetes. *Diabetes Care* 2009;32:1947–1953

54. Hirsch I, et al. Clinical application of emerging sensor technologies in diabetes management: consensus guidelines for continuous glucose monitoring. *Diabetes Technol Ther* 2008;10(4):232–244

55. Evert A, Trence D, Catton S, Huynh P. Continuous glucose monitoring technology for personal use: an educational program that educates and supports the patient. *Diabetes Educator* 2009;35(4):565–580

56. Raccah D, et al. Incremental value of continuous glucose monitoring when starting pump therapy in patients with poorly controlled type 1 diabetes: the RealTrend study. *Diabetes Care* 2009;32(12):2245–2250

57. Bohnett L, et al. Increased continuous glucose monitoring (CGM) receiver interaction is associated with glycemic benefit in pediatric patients. *Cureus* 2012;4(9):e13

Index

Note: Page numbers followed by *t* refer to tables. Page numbers followed by *f* refer to figures. Page numbers in **bold** indicate an in-depth discussion on the topic.

A

absolute difference, 10*t*
accident, 34
acetaminophen, 19, 88
active insulin time, 63
activities, 67–72
adhesion, 13, 77, 82–83, 86
air travel, 84
alcohol, 34, 48
alert, 3, 6–8, 13, 25–33, 79–80, 90
allergy, 82
American Diabetes Association
    Standards of Care, 44
amylin, 66, 91
ancillary transmission equipment, 8
Android phone, 9
angry bolus, 30
Animas Vibe insulin pump, 6

applications (apps), 8, 68, 72
artificial pancreas, 33, 91

B

baby monitor, 80
Band-Aid Tough Pad, 82
battery, 13
Bergenstal, R., 35
biguanide, 56
birth weight, 14
blood glucose (BG). *See
    also* hyperglycemia;
    hypoglycemia
    accuracy, 10–12
    alternate site reading, 78
    bolus adjustment, 23–25
    calibration values, 7
    data, 39
    fingerstick glucose monitoring, 49

lag time, 11–12, 27
point-in-time reading, 3
postmeal, 29
predictive alert, 32
premeal, 29
real-time information, 17–19
standard deviation, 43–44
target range, 44–46
trend arrow, 6
Bluetooth, 8
buttock, 81

C

Cal Factor, 88
calibration, 7, 11–13, 18–19, 40–41, 49, 78–81, 88–89
calorie, 42
carbohydrate, 21–23, 27, 30–32, 34, 39, 50, 56
case study, **48–75**
cause-and-effect relationship, 15, 40
CGM Anti-Denial Campaign, 85
CGM in the Cloud, 9
children, 9, 14, 45
closed loop system, 33
cloud-based server, 8–9
Compeed Moisture Seal technology, 82
continuous glucose monitoring (CGM)
   accuracy, 10–13
   benefits, 2, **17–34**
   candidates recommended for usage, 14–15

data analysis, **35–75**
decision making, 20–21
device specific challenges, 86–89
downsides of, **77–91**
essentials of, **3–15**
old-school CGM system, 19*f*
personal system, 43
professional use systems, 41–42
real-time, maximizing the benefits in, **17–34**
Contour Next Link USB meter, 38–39
control solution, 79
correction factor, 56–58
cost, 78, 84–85
cost-to-benefit ratio, 14
counter-regulatory responses, 27

D

data
   analysis, **35–75**
   ancillary transmission equipment, 8
   context, 42
   decision making tool, 3–4
   evaluation of, 90
   inaccuracy, 11–12, 41
   lag time, 11–12
   qualification, 40–41
   receivers and displays, 6
   skipped, 84
   software, 7
delayed onset hypoglycemia, 69

Dexcom
  acetaminophen, 19
  ancillary transmission
      equipment, 8
  bolus adjustment, 24t
  calibration, 79
  charging cable, 89
  continuous glucose monitoring,
      4
  Glucose Trend report, 64, 73–74
  insurance plan resources, 85
  maintenance, 13
  Patterns report, 54
  real-time information, 17
  receiver, 6, 88–89
  sensor adhesive, 83
  software, 36t
  transmitter, 88
  trend, 20t
  trend graph, 53, 60, 66–72
Dexcom Diasend, 7, 36t, 38
Dexcom G4 Professional system, 4,
    11t, 88–89
Dexcom G4 SHARE, 9
Dexcom SHARE, 8–9
Dexcom Studio software, 7, 36–38,
    41, 46f, 49–51
diabetes education, 32, 75, 78
diabetes management, 3, 75, 85, 90
dipeptidyl peptidase-4 inhibitors, 56
display, 6, 8
durable medical equipment, 84–85

E
elderly, 45t
electrical power/current, 5–6, 13
equipment, 4–5
essentials, 4–15
event marker, 42, 68
exercise, 20, 21t, 30, 56, 68, 75, 90

F
fast, 42
FDA (U.S. Food and Drug
    Administration), 4–5, 18,
    30, 81
fingerstick glucose monitoring
    accuracy, 10–11
    alcohol swab, 78
    alternate site reading, 78
    calibration, 79
    cleanliness, 78
    glucose meter, 78
    hypoglycemia, 19, 27, 30–31, 47
    point-in-time glucose readings, 3
    result confirmation, 79
    sensor calibration, 7
    vs. sensor glucose, 18–19, 49
    Thresh Suspend alert, 88

G
gestational diabetes, 45t
glargine, 60, 64, 71–72
glucagon, 56, 91
glucagon-like peptide-1 (GLP-1)
    analog, 56, 66
glucose meter, 78–79

glucose response curve, 63
glucose value, 17–19, 37, 44
glycemic control, 14–15
glycosuria, 57

H

HbA$_{1c}$, 14, 35, 85
health care provider, 4, 18, 32, 38–39, 78, 82
health professional organizations, 14
heart disease, 45t
HemoCue, 11t
high/low alert, 7, 12, 25–32, 34, 40, 80
hormonal change, 47
hormone-delivery device, 91
hydrocolloidal dressing, 82
hyperglycemia, 3, 7, 26, 33, 40, 63–66, 73
hypoglycemia. *See also* severe hypoglycemia
    alcohol, 34
    alert/alert settings, 3, 7, 80–81
    basal settings test, 43
    CGM use, regular, 89
    correction factor, 58
    delayed onset, 69
    exercise, 69
    fingerstick glucose monitoring, 19, 27, 30–31, 47
    high/low alert, 25–31
    low shut-off feature, 33
    Medtronic CareLink Pro, 40
    overtreatment, 65

pattern, 47–48, 74
predictive alert, 32
pregnancy, 14
rate-of-change alert, 31
sensor glucose data, 43
treatment, 21–22, 64–66
trend graph, 22
hypoglycemia unawareness, 14, 25–26, 33–34, 45, 85

I

illness, 56, 90
incretin mimetics, 66–67
infection, 81
inflammation, 81
insertion device, 4, 5f
insulin
    action curve, 62–64
    aspart, 64
    basal, 7, 33–34, 39, 42–43, 59–63, 74–75, 88
    bolus, 23–25, 39, 75
    bolus-on-board, 30
    bolus sculpting, 52
    dose magnitude, 53
    glucose sensor data, 91
    hypoglycemia unawareness, 26
    injection, 42
    low/high alert, 27
    mealtime dose, 53–56
    peak, 52t
    post-correction bolus, 30
    rapid-acting, 23–25, 30–31, 50, 60

sensitivity, 24, 56–58

sensor glucose decision making, 21

insulin-on-board (IOB), 26, 30, 62–63, 90

insulin pump, 6–7, 13, 23–25, 33

insulin pump therapy, 40, 42, 62–63, 73–74, 82, 88, 91

insulin-to-carbohydrate ratio, 54, 56

insurance, 14, 78, 84–85, 91

intensive diabetes management, 14–15

International Organization for Standardization, 18

interstitial-fluid-between-the-fat-cells glucose concentration, 18

iPhone, 8

iPod Touch, 8

irritation, 83

IV3000, 82–83

J

JDRF, 85, 89

K

ketone, 32

L

lab glucose value, 10t–11t

lag time, 11–13, 18–19, 27, 29, 43, 65, 77–79

letter sample, 85

lifestyle event, 67–72, 75

liraglutide, 66–67

log, 42, 68, 72

low shut-off feature, 33–34

M

macrosomia, 14

magnetic resonance imaging (MRI) equipment, 84

Mahony, Jon, 28f

maintenance, 13

mean (average), 43

mean absolute difference (MAD) percentage, 41

mean absolute relative difference percentage (MARD%), 10, 11t

medication, 15, 56, 90. See also under specific type

Medtronic

 ancillary transmission equipment, 8

 bolus adjustment, 24t

 continuous glucose monitoring, 4

 insulin pump, 39, 58, 84

 maintenance, 13

 needle housing, 87f

 pump automation, 33

 real-time information, 17

 receiver, 6–7

 reimbursement guide for health care professionals, 85

 sensor, 33

 Sof-sensor, 6

 software, 36t

 trend, 20t

Medtronic 530G insulin pump, 6–7, 33

Medtronic CareLink, 7, 36t, 38–39, 41, 45, 46f, 63

Medtronic CareLink Pro, 7, 36t, 39–40, 46, 51–52, 54, 58–59, 65, 73

Medtronic CareLink USB, 38–39

Medtronic Enlite, 4, 11t, 83–84, 86–88

Medtronic Enlite Serter, 87f

Medtronic Guardian, 6, 13, 84

Medtronic iPro Professional system, 4, 13

Medtronic MiniLink, 13

Medtronic mySentry, 8

Medtronic Veo, 33

menses, 70–71

meter capillary glucose, 11t

meter value, 10t

MiniMed CGMS, 70

mobile device, 8–9

modal-day trend graph, 46

N

needle housing, 87f

NightScout, 9

numeric value report, 11–12

O

OPSITE FLEXFIX, 83

oral hypoglycemic agent, 26, 49–50

out-of-pocket cost, 84–85

P

pattern, 36–37, 39, 47–48, 52t, 55, 90

pattern report, **46–75**

Pearson, I., 35

percentage adjustment, 24–25

percent difference, 10

performance, 10–11

physical activity, 21, 30, 39

point-in-time glucose reading, 3

postmeal excursion, 50

postmeal peak, 50, 75

postprandial spike, 50–53

postprandial trend analysis, 40

pramlintide, 56

predictive alert, 7, 26, 32–33, 80

pregnancy, 14, 59

preparation, 41–46

professional use system, 4

pump automation, 33–34

R

radio frequency, 6

radio signal, 11

radio transmitter, 5

rate-of-change alert, 7, 26, 31–32, 80

real-time information, 6, **17–34**, 90

real-time system, 4

reception/receiver, 6, 13, 77, 84, 90–91

report, 37. *See also under specific type*

rise-rate alert, 73

rotation chart, 81, 82t

S

scar tissue, 81
sensitivity, 82
sensor
    alcohol swab, 86
    alert, 40
    alert fatigue, 73
    essential equipment, 4–5
    false alarm, 77
    graph, 47
    inaccuracy, 11–13, 77
    insertion device, 77, 81, 86–87
    lag time, 11–13, 77
    maintenance, 13
    rocker motion, 86
    site management, 81
    statistical data, 46f
    storage, 86
    tracing, 57
sensor glucose (SG)
    critical decision making, 18–19
    data, 38–39, 43, 49–50
    Dexcom Studio software, 41
    hypoglycemia, 22f, 23
    lag time, 27, 29
    low/high alert, 27–28
    low shut-off feature, 34
    mean (average), 43
    Medtronic CareLink Pro, 40
    pattern analysis, 38–39
    trend, 7, 20–23
    value, 7
sensor-triggered intervention, 27

severe hypoglycemia, 26–27, 33–34, 45, 45t
shenanigans, 72–74
signal loss, 84
site management, 81–84
skin irritation, 12
smartphone app, 68, 80, 91
sodium-glucose transporter-2inhibitor, 57
software, 7, 35–46
standard deviation, 43–44
steroid medication, 57, 82
strategies for success, 89–90
stress, 56, 70
subcutaneous fat, 81

T

target range, 44–46
technology, 1–3, 7, 89–91
Tegaderm, 82–83
test, 42–43
test strip, 78–79
thiazolidinediones, 56
threshold suspend feature, 33
Thresh Suspend alert, 88
transmission/transmitter, 5–9, 13, 77, 84, 86–88
trend, 19–25, 90
trend arrow, 20t–21t, 23–25
trend graph, **46–75**
    case study, 20, 21t, 24–26, 66–67, 70–71
    communicating, 60
    individual-day, 64–65

metallic connector, 86
postprandial spike, 50–52
real-time information, 6
report, 11
type 1 diabetes, 26, 45t, 49, 85
type 2 diabetes, 26, 45t, 49, 85

U

user guide specification, 11t
U.S. Food and Drug Administration.
    See FDA

V

venous serum glucose, 10
vibratory alert, 6–7

W

walkie-talkie, 80
web-based program, 7
web resources, 85

Y

Yellow Springs Instrument (YSI), 10,
    11t